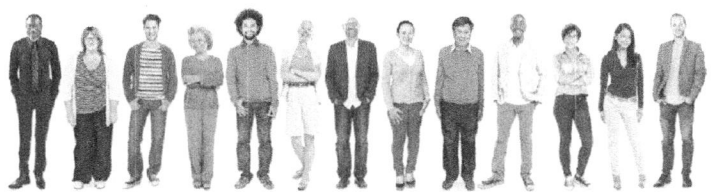

REASONABLE EXPECTATIONS:
The Patient Side of Patient Centered Care

A BOOK BY

De'Andre Alexander | Aaliyah Anaya
Olivia Arkell | Riham Alwaely
Hugo Amador | Abigail Arient
Emelia Behnan | Julianna Celestin
Dima Bischoff-Hashem
Airiana Michelle Davis | Anat Ferleger
Bansi Kakadiya | Bansari Kheni
Bob Kieserman | Mason La Fleur
Juhi Patel | Yu-Tung (Anna) Lu
Courtney Pokallus | Michelle Powell
Regina Rush | Anooshka Shukla
Tasfia Wahid | Faalik Zahra

ROBERT H. KIESERMAN, EDITOR

Copyright © 2022 by Robert H. Kieserman

All rights reserved. No part of this book may be reproduced or used in any manner without the prior written permission of the copyright owner, except for the use of brief quotations in a book review.

To request permissions, contact the publisher at powerofpatient@gmail.com

Paperback: 9798846711341

First paperback edition September 2022

Printed by MedFocus Publications in the United States of America

The Power of the Patient Project:
The National Library of Patient Rights and Advocacy
Cherry Hill, New Jersey 08002

www.thepowerofthepatient.org

PAGE

INTRODUCTION   *5*

PART ONE: DEFINITIONS
1. What is Patient Centered Care?   10
2. What are the Social Determinants of Health?   24

PART TWO: THE INFLUENCERS
3. The Providers   33
4. The Support Staff   40
5. The Administrators   44
6. Healthcare Facilities   51

PART THREE: THE INFLUENCES
7. The Patient's Education   60
8. The Patient's Gender   67
9. The Patient's Socioeconomic Status   76
10. Where a Patient Lives   82
11. The Patient's Social Circle   89
12. The Patient's Access to Healthcare   93
13 The Right of Self-Determination   101

PART FOUR: LIFE CYCLES
14. Birth to Adolescence   110
15. Young Adult   117
16. Middle Age   120
17. Senior Years   126
18. End of Life   135

PART FIVE: STRENGTHS AND THREATS
19. The Impact of Communication   153
20. The Impact of Corporate Medicine   161
21. Is Patient Centered Care Working?   168

About the Authors   174

INTRODUCTION

This is a book about expectations. Everyone has them. About all kinds of things. We have things we would like to see happen for ourselves, our families, our friends, and for others. Sometimes these expectations are met, and sometimes they are not. When they are met, we feel gratified and all is well in our world, but when they are not, it is normal to be disappointed, perhaps even frustrated.

Patients are no exception. Patients have expectations and they are reasonable expectations. Patients have expectations of their providers, their healthcare insurance company, their hospitals, and the healthcare delivery system in general. We expect our providers to be the best doctors and therapists they can possibly be, up to date on the research, and patient-friendly. When we have a doctor or therapist who shows compassion and has earned our trust, we feel great about the relationship, and know we are in the best of hands. When we need to go the emergency room or need to be hospitalized, we expect the experience to be a positive one where the doctors and nurses and all of the support staff are showing compassion and paying complete attention to our needs in our moment of a health crisis.

However, sometimes the compassion and the complete attention is missing, and when those things do not seem to be happening, we begin to have doubts about our care.

I spent much of my career educating future healthcare administrators and future providers, preparing my students to manage hospitals, nursing homes, ambulatory care centers, urgent care centers, and medical practices. I also helped others to prepare to enter the healthcare professions as future physicians, nurses, rehab therapists, mental health therapists, and physician assistants. As a professor of healthcare administration and medical ethics, my focus was on teaching the business of medicine.

My ultimate goal was to reinforce to my students the importance of always fostering the best patient experience possible.

In 2017, several of my students at that time and I collaborated to create The Power of the Patient Project, a digital library focused on empowering patients about their rights and fostering a better relationship with their providers. A year later, we deemed the Project the National Library of Patient Rights and Advocacy through the National Library of Medicine in Bethesda, Maryland. Little did I know at the time that the Project would gain an international following and become a major information resource for thousands of patients. It is my passion for a positive patient experience that prompted the creation of this book.

Patient Centered Care
For years, providers and healthcare facilities along with their professional associations have advocated for something called patient centered care. Patient centered care has many dimensions, and is rooted in expectations.

This book is about the expectations of patients regarding patient centered care.

Some people might ask, why do we need to write a book about patient centered care? After all, isn't all the care we receive from our doctors and other healthcare providers always patient centered? That would be assumed. Right? Well, quite frankly, I find myself becoming more and more concerned that it is not always the case anymore.

Patient or Profit
This book will explore whether patient centered care is really being practiced as well as it should. My concern is whether hospitals and medical practices are truly dedicated to providing the best care possible with a focus on the patient, or if they are really more concerned with the financial bottom

line. With the growth of for-profit companies owning and operating hospitals and physician practices, something that has been labeled *corporate medicine,* my concern has become even greater in the past few years. Much to my dismay, there are still few medical schools in the country including a course on patient centered care in their program. When a hospital or other healthcare facility advertises for a new doctor or administrator, there are not too many ads that mention patient centered care. This causes me concern, and that is why we are writing this book, to explore the true status of this noble goal called patient centered care.

How the Book is Structured for the Reader
This book is exploring patient centered care using the principles of the Social Determinants of Health as its basis. In 2003, the World Health Organization (WHO) provided the medical sociology community with a set of guidelines to "provide a deep understanding of health disparities in a global perspective". In Part One of the book, **Definitions**, the first chapter defines patient centered care and Chapter Two is devoted to explaining the Social Determinants of Health for the reader.

The chapters that follow in Part Two address the men and women who provide the healthcare, the providers, as well as those who support the providers in our hospitals, urgent care centers, surgical centers, and healthcare practices. You probably know the second group as the folks at the front desk, the receptionists, medical assistants, and administrators. We call them **The Influencers**, because all of the providers and all of those who support their work directly affect the patient experience.

Part Three looks at the expectations of patients from each of the Social Determinants of Health, and how that affects the patient's perception of quality care. This section examines **The Influences**. How does a patient's education or the social circle of the patient or how much access to care a patient has affected their expectations as a patient?

The chapters in Part Four then look at **Life Cycles of the Patient** and how our expectations of patient centered care change throughout our lives.

Finally, the final section, Part Five, **The Strengths and Weaknesses**, explores the important role of Patient/Provider Relations, the impact of corporate medicine, and concludes with an assessment of whether patient centered care is working and truly benefiting the practice experience.

It is our hope that you will enjoy the book and learn from its pages. We have purposely written the book using a reader-friendly approach.

I have been joined in this endeavor by a team of co-authors who are talented researchers and writers from a variety of backgrounds in science, public health, and healthcare administration. I have also been assisted throughout the writing of this book by Courtney Pokallus, who assumed the role of Project Manager and co-authored several chapters with me. This has been a superb experience for me working with these bright, young professionals, who have so much insight into the patient experience. All of us are dedicated to ensuring that the patient experience is always a positive experience. Thank you for joining us as we explore this very important aspect of all of our lives.

Bob Kieserman
Fall, 2022

PART ONE
DEFINITIONS

Chapter One

What is Patient Centered Care?
By Riham Alwaely, Emelia Behnan, and Yu-Tung (Anna) Lu

Definition of Patient Centered Care
So, let's start at the very beginning. How do we define patient centered care? As you will see, it is defined in many different ways by different stakeholders in patient care. So to begin, we want to introduce you to several healthcare providers, several healthcare administrators, and several major healthcare organizations to hear what they have to say and how they define patient centered care.

We are so fortunate in this country to have probably the best healthcare system in the world. Overseeing our healthcare system is a large network of government agencies at the federal level, state level, and local level, starting with the Department of Health and Human Services in Washington, D.C.. However, the independent professional organizations that oversee our hospitals and other facilities, our medical practices, and our providers also have tremendous impact on the care that patients receive, and so it makes sense to start with them.

The Professional Organizations
So. how do the major professional organizations define patient centered care?

The American Medical Association, one of the major professional associations in this country, and the organization that advocates for and educates physicians and to which most doctors in this country belong, provides this definition:

"Patient-centered care is the practice of assessing patient-centered care through the lens of care coordination and patient satisfaction."

The American Hospital Association, the organization that oversees the hospitals in this country, defines it as:

"Comprehensive care that meets the large majority of each patient's physical and mental health care needs, including prevention and wellness, acute care, and chronic care. Patient-centered care that is relationship-based with an orientation toward the whole person".

The American Nursing Association, the organization that oversees the nursing profession, defines it as:

"Patient-centered care coordination is a core professional standard for all registered nurses and is central to nurses' longtime practice of providing holistic care to patients—incorporating interventions from a variety of disciplines into traditional health care approaches."

The American College of Healthcare Executives, the organization that oversees the integrity and professional excellence of the men and women who manage the country's healthcare facilities, defines it in this way:

"Care that is respectful of and responsive to individual patient preferences, needs, and values, and ensuring that patient values guide all clinical decisions."

The American Dental Association, the organzation that oversees the practice of dentistry, defines patient centered care as "delivering dental care services that make sense to our patients, that are patient friendly and that reconcile the common barriers to care. These barriers can be summarized under the following themes – fear, trust, time, cost and value."

The Picker Institute
And finally, The Picker Insitute, which is described as "a world leader focusing on the measurement of the patient experience and recognized as an important source of information, advice and support. The board of directors supports the advancement of the science through programs, research and awards that recognize "best practices," all designed to foster a continued improvement in healthcare from the patient's perspective … through the patient's eyes. The Gold Foundation supports the development and dissemination of innovative medical education that furthers this mission. The Picker Institute sponsors education and research in the field of patient-centered care in cooperation with educational institutions and other interested entities and individuals. The institute's goal is to foster a broader understanding of the practical and theoretical implications of patient-centered care by approaching healthcare with a focus on the concerns of patients and other healthcare consumers."

The Picker Institute defines patient centered care as "the practice of caring for patients (and their families) in ways that are meaningful and valuable to the individual patient. It includes listening to, informing and involving patients in their care."

The Basic Themes of the Definitions
So, what are the basic themes that we see in the definitions of the professional associations? First, assessing what patients expect, and then striving for patient satisfaction, creating a bond between the patient and the provider, aspiring to the highest standards of caring for patients, and ensuring that the values of patients guide clinical decisions. To us as patients, these principles of practice sound like a ideal patient centered care model.

The Providers
But how about the providers themselves? Do the providers buy into this model set by their professional associations? Let's take a look at some feedback from a representative group of healthcare providers to see.

Lindsay Tobey, OTR/L
Lindsay Tobey is a licensed registered occupational therapist who specializes in hand therapy. To Lindsay, who treats a wide range of patients of all ages, "Patient centered care is not just about understanding a patient's diagnosis and knowing how to treat it."

As she further explains it, "While that is an important aspect, it shouldn't be at the forefront of patient centered care. The most important aspect of patient centered care is building rapport. As an occupational therapist, the first thing we do at an evaluation is build an occupational profile. Using the guidelines of The American Occupational Therapy Association, the occupational profile is a summary of a client's occupational history and experiences, patterns of daily living, interests, values, needs, and relevant contexts. We see the whole person before we see the diagnosis. Occupational therapy is all about getting the patient back to doing what they love doing whether it be playing a sport, going back to work, or participating in other hobbies. Improving the patient's range of motion and strength is an important aspect of hand therapy, but patients will feel more cared for and get better results when you take the time to get to know them. Let them know that you are a team and you are working together to build a therapy program to get them back to their prior level of functioning. Building rapport doesn't end right after evaluation. Patient centered care continues throughout the entire therapy process. It is important to continue to build rapport throughout the patient's plan of care and remembering the little details about their life. When you remember the little things, it makes a big impact on their motivation to come to therapy. Patients shouldn't feel like they are just a reimbursement or profit. Patient centered care is all about making the patient feel comfortable, competent in your skills to treat, and well cared for."

Danielle Ofri, MD, PhD

Dr. Danille Ofri is a world-renown physician and author of eight best-selling books. Her book, *What Patients Say, What Doctors Hear* is the classic book on exploring the provider/patient relationship. She very much believes and practices patient centered care, but she explains what can unfortunately compromise that relationship.

"The system seems to work against it and I'll start with the issue of time so when I see my patients in a lot of 10 or 15 minutes. If a patient is completely healthy and there for a checkup, that window of time works. But if a patient has five or six chronic issues, chronic illness, a psychological challenge, stress or depression, or perhaps food insecurity or financial insecurity, we need to talk about it, and it may not take just 15 minutes. Maybe the patient does not speak English and we need to use an interpreter to have our dialogue, and maybe that patient is taking 18 different medications. I can spend the entire visit just sorting through that and will never have a chance to get to know them, who they live with, what is their circumstance, how they came to this country, what they do for a living all these things are so important. What's important to you in life, those things are critical to understanding the patient and without enough time that's one of the hardest things I face as a doctor."

Paul Kaloostian, M.D.

Dr. Paul Kaloostian is a neurosurgeon and one of the country's major patient advocates whose medical practice is a model for optimal patient centered care. Here is what he says about upholding a strong patient/provider relationship:

"What are some things that will improve the experience patients have when visiting their doctor? I always think sitting down with a patient versus a doctor standing up is a starting point. I know myself as a patient with my doctor sitting down with me as opposed to just running around the room and trying to leave is very disturbing. I think the doctor sitting down calms the patient down. The power of touch I think is also very important and there's nothing worse than a doctor that doesn't even look at you or touch you. I think that distances that relationship and makes the outcome worse so I think an examination is very important. With the power of touch, there's that energy transferred between two human beings and it shows the patient that the provider is really interested in finding out what's going on. We need to show the patient that we care about the patient and we want to help the patient. And finally, empathy for the patient means everything. We need to repeat what the patient is saying to us, so we can convince the patient that look, I am listening to you, I hear what you are saying, and I need you to have a conversation with me so I can better diagnose you and help you."

Christopher R. Westfall, DMD

Dr. Christopher Westfall is a highly respected general dentist practicing in Southern New Jersey. His practice is recognized for its focus on patient centered care. According to Dr. Westfall, "patient centered care is an overt acknowledgment of patient first care. It is important to not only hear our patients, but to listen to their goals, needs, wants, and wishes. This may in fact be quite different from our assessment and subjective summary of the patient's condition. When the patient is educated and informed, the treatment plan may serve as an objective path of departure that is validated by the patient. The plan can then involve integrated care that may include family and trusted friends. This blueprint will help our patients to navigate the complex journey that they face. This voyage, however, may seem a little more manageable if the care is patient driven. Perhaps, we may see more success knowing that the care is being rendered and ultimately driven by the patients themselves!"

Logan Nester, DPT

Dr. Logan Nester is a physical therapist who specializes in pelvic health. Her patients are women and also some men who are experiencing embarrasing medical conditions that come with age and for other reasons, so her approach must be compassionate and very patient centered. She comments on the impact of the financial considerations that many patients have and how that becomes part of the equation when talking about patient centered care.

"I've had the opportunity to experience both insurance-based and cash-based physical therapy care, which has given me substantial perspective. Insurance-based therapy, which can be more convenient, inclusive regarding financial disposition, and sometimes more cost effective depending on the case or severity, sadly can provide less quality care compared to a cash-based therapy practice, in my opinion. Insurance unfortunately provides a progressive burden, unfair reimbursement, less one on one care, and often, the patient's access to care. At the same time, in order to stay open, physical therapy offices must see as many patients in a week as they can, which directly impacts patient care. Unfortunately this model is highly associated with clinician burnout, often causing good clinicians to leave the profession. Although it can be a great challenge for physical therapists to continue to provide quality care, we must remember that the patients are victims of this broken system and we must do our best to provide them with a good experience and tools to continue their recovery beyond financial, insurance, and prognosis constraints."

"In my opinion, although many patients question this approach, cash-based therapy is a better approach to ensure patient centered care because it better allows therapists to provide one on one care that is actually more appropriate for the patient in the short and the long term."

"We must be the therapists we want for ourselves. Most of us take pride in the time we are able to spend with patients, understanding their backgrounds and constructing the most comprehensive and customized care - which is a very unique sector of health care. Physical therapy is truly an art more than it is a science - we have the time, power, and influencing body to create optimal, patient-centered care. Although reimbursement greatly impacts our day to day care and sometimes the progress of the patient, we must take the extra time to create a positive, patient-centered experience."

The Administrators

Thousands of men and women across the country work in our nation's healthcare facilities as the administrators. Trained to manage the business of healthcare, they oversee the operations of hospitals, nursing homes, assisted living communities, medical practices, urgent care centers, ambulatory surgical centers, and many other related facilities. They have their own perception of patient centered care. Here is just a sampling to allow you to understand the important perspective they bring to your healthcare.

Michael Cahill, LNHA

Michael Cahill is licensed nursing home administrator and the administrator of a large skilled nursing inpatient facility in Philadelphia. He believes that "No two patients are alike. It is our role as the administrators of a healthcare facility to strive to meet the preferences of the patient and to always protect the patient. We cannot ever forget the importance of the family, and that a supportive and loving family greatly supports the recovery of the patient. That is the essence of patient centered care".

Beth Duffy

Beth Duffy is President and Chief Operating Officer of Einstein Montgomery Hospital, a part of Einstein Healthcare Network/Jefferson Health in a suburb of Philadelphia. She believes that patient centered care can best be defined as "looking at the whole patient based on their specific healthcare needs and desired outcomes. When we built our facility ten years ago, we incorporated patient centered care aspects as we built it. We also use feedback from our patient experience surveys to drive change. We use our patient experience surveys as a main way of gathering information. From the day we opened our facility, our approach has always been patient centered care. It matters to us very much, and it matters to the patient even more".

Dwight McBee
Dwight McBee is Executive Vice President for Health Health Equity and Patient and Family Experience at Jefferson Health in Philadelphia. Simply stated, he offers the approach of this world renown hospital system as "an approach to the planning, delivery, and evaluation of health care that is grounded in mutually beneficial partnerships among healthcare providers, patients, and families. In short, we don't want to do anything concerning our patients without feedback from our patients."

"We respect the unique needs and preferences of our patients and families and strive to create a system of care delivery to support the greatest level of wellness for those we serve. Our approach to delivering healthcare is based on the core principles of dignity, respect, information sharing, participation and collaboration".

The Patients
And how about patients? How do patients view patient centered care? More importantly, how do you personally see it? What is important to you when you enter a hospital for treatment or you visit with a doctor, a therapist, or a mental health counselor?

Most patients agree that closeness to the provider's office is really important. No one wants to drive further than they need to, especially when they are not feeling well. So, many patients who depend on public transportation value when a hospital or doctor's office is accessible by bus, cab, train, or subway. At the same time, patients who are driving value the accommodation of a parking area to make the visit easier. Patients value the ease of making an appointment with their primary care physician or specialists when they need an appointment, and value the ability to get through to a live person who can make the appointment for them. Because many insurance plans require referrals to specialists, patients also value clear instructions provided on when and how to get referrals.

At the same time, most patients believe that patient centered care is being practiced by a hospital or medical office when there is *shared decision-making*, giving patients, the families of patients, and caretakers a say in the care plan decisions and giving them time to research before making those decisions. We as patients also expect customized care, being treated as a unique individual who deserves to choose from multiple diagnostic and treatment options. We also value information sharing, where we are presented with all the observations and data the care team has gathered, as well as the latest relevant condition and treatment research upon which we can make smart and educated decisions about our healthcare options.

So, How Do We Evaluate the Care We Receive?
The medical profession evaluates patient centered care by whether expected outcomes are met. Was the patient satisfied with their visit and experience, with how well they healed, with the cost efficiency, and more. To put it in defined terms, this evaluation measures efficiency, effectiveness, satisfaction, and equity.

But how do we as patients evaluate our healthcare experience in terms of what is important to us? What are our reasonable expectations of our providers, of our healthcare facilities, or our insurance companies, and of the healthcare delivery system in general?

Most patients will answer the question with several key priorities. Patients want to feel respected. Patients want to be heard. Patients want to feel trusted and they want to be able to trust their providers and those caring for them in a hospital. Patients want to be treated as individuals - coming from different cultures, ethnic groups, gender orientations, age groups, religions, different neighborhoods, with different life experiences, and different outlooks on life. We value when a provider listens to us with an open mind acknowledging our point of view, and when they value a family member or friend being part of the visit, to serve as a second pair of ears for us. We value when a provider takes time to read our emotions and offers the emotional support we need, especially when we are suffering with pain, upset by a possible diagnosis, scared of the future, or simply stressed out.

We, as patients, evaluate the care we receive by how well those providing the care pay attention to our expectations and how well the providers integrate those things into caring for us medically. We all know how easy it is to feel like simply a number. Patient centered care needs to be practiced with the focus on us, who we are and what each of us is all about.

In the next chapter of the book, we will explore the Social Determinants of Health, those factors that contribute to our health, but are not necessarily biological in nature. Factors such as where we live, where we work and what we do, our educational background, our age, our gender, our economic stability, our access to healthcare, and the level of community we experience all affect our overall health and very much affect optimal patient centered care.

Chapter Two

What are the Social Determinants of Health?

By Riham Alwaely, Julianna Celestin, Regina Rush, Anooshka Shukla, Olivia Arkell, and Bansari Kheni

We know that the biological functions of our bodies control our health. When everything in our body is working properly and doing what it is supposed to do, we are well, and feel good. We also know that regular exercise, healthy eating, reducing stress, and laughing a lot improves our health and helps the biological functions to work at their optimum. But there are some important other factors that also directly affect our overall health and wellbeing. These factors are known as the Social Determinants of Health, and their effect on our emotional stability greatly influences the biological functions of our body, and therefore, our overall health. Scientists are now convinced that these other factors have a direct effect on how we feel, how we age, and how we function.

What are Social Determinants of Health?
The Social Determinants of Health are the non-medical factors that influence health outcomes. These are the societal circumstances in which individuals are born into, live, and grow. Factors such as economic stability, educational access and quality, the environment, our access to healthcare and quality of care, where we work, our home life, how much stress we have in our life, our age, and our social network all affect our wellbeing. An individual's socioeconomic status, their cost of living, house stability, and food security all pay a role in their health.

Addressing the Social Determinants of Health is important for improving health outcomes and reducing longstanding disparities in health care.

The Role of Culture on the Social Determinants
Culture is a foundational determinant of health. According to the Office of Minority Health of the United States Department of Health and Human Services, culture is the unique shared values, beliefs, and practices that a group of patients share, based on where they live, their religion, or what has been passed down from generation to generation in their family structure. Culture is an important determinant of an individual's perception of illness/ diseases. Some patients may have different beliefs when it comes to the cause of their disease/illness and how they contracted the illness/disease. Moreover, culture influences health choices for individuals. This includes choosing the right physicians, which professionals to trust, and which primary doctor to believe in and confide in.

The American Culture
American culture acknowledges that there are different cultures. However, health related practices and behaviors, both in past and present, are not inclusive to all cultures. They are significantly aligned to and catered to "American culture". Meaning, White/Caucasian men and women. This is called *cultural hegemony*, which is essentially when the dominant group of a culturally diverse society, typically the privileged and ruling class, manipulates the culture of that society.

Meaning the preeminent culture influences their considered beliefs and reasoning, perceptions, morals, etc. so that their viewpoints develop into the "affirmed" cultural norm. The "American culture" sets the standards of care. This is significantly illustrated in how healthcare professionals treat cultures and racial/ethnic groups in our healthcare system. In the *International Journal for Equity in Health*, it is cited that particular groups may receive poorer standards of care due to biased beliefs or attitudes held by health professionals. The hegemonic culture of America has resulted in the mistreatment, misdiagnosis, racial bias, and discrimination of racial/ethnic communities.

Accessibility to Nutritious Food

There is no question that nutritious food is a staple for good health. One of the biggest problems in this country is that there are many people who do not have proper and adequate access to good nutritious food. One of the primary reasons for a lack of accessibility to food is *supermarket redlining*. Supermarket redlining is when major supermarket chains and corporations choose not to locate their stores in inner cities, rural and urban low socioeconomic neighborhoods. According to the United States Department of Agriculture Economic Research Service, supermarket redlining intentionally results in local residents lacking stores that sell and adequately provide healthy and affordable food alternatives. Supermarket redlining is a reason why people living in low socioeconomic areas find it challenging to gain access to fresh and quality groceries and pay higher prices for groceries. For this reason, inadequate access to fresh and quality groceries in these impoverished areas contributes the residents to diet-related illnesses like obesity, diabetes, high blood pressure, and poor nutrition. When good food is not readily available, we say that these folks are living in *food deserts*.

Food deserts are geographical areas where it is difficult to buy healthy, nutritious food at an affordable price. In communities across the United States, there are approximately 23.5 million people who are living in locations known as food deserts. A study published by the *Journal of the American Heart Association* concluded that individuals living in food deserts have a significantly greater risk of heart disease. A 2021 study conducted by Tulane University emphasized that people living in food deserts who frequently rely on fast food for their main meals are seven times more at risk of having a stroke before the age of 45, double the possible risks of a heart attack and Type 2 diabetes, and four times as likely to be at risk for kidney failure. These vulnerable residents are being bombarded with a double-ended sword; not being able to acquire affordable healthy foods while being presented with access to unhealthy and affordable food.

Supermarket Distance and Food Swamps
Published studies have shown evidence that within low socioeconomic neighborhoods, residents living in areas with an increasing proportion of African American/Black and Latino populations have to travel longer distances to their nearest supermarket. Studies have shown that on average, in predominantly African American and Latino neighborhoods, people need to travel approximately one to 1.25 more miles to the nearest supermarket than neighborhoods with predominantly white populations, and that prominently white neighborhoods had four times more supermarkets within a reasonable traveling distance than prominently non-white neighborhoods. The bottom line is that the fast food restaurant companies often focus on placing their restaurants in low income neighborhoods. Sociologists call these food swamps.

Food swamps are conventionally described as specific areas with a high density of local establishments that sell and promote high-calorie fortified food and junk food, compared to healthier food options. Fast food companies intentionally take advantage of these people and their vulnerable situations in order to make a profit. Meanwhile, these companies are intentionally selling inexpensive meals that traditionally incorporate processed meats and dairy-based foods high in saturated fats, fructose corn syrup, and sodium, and therefore, this contributes to the poor health of these low income populations.

Housing, Neighborhood, and Physical Environment

Many individuals are very surprised to learn that our neighborhood, where we live, also has a great effect on our health.

Families who have greater access to safe and stable housing tend to have easy access to affordable fruits and vegetables, and can easily access safe open spaces where they can be physically active, giving them better health outcomes. Low socioeconomic neighborhoods frequently lack nutritious food and ideal living conditions that are needed to adequately support a healthy lifestyle. If one's environment has inadequate resources, has physical and social barriers, and the people who reside there are not financially stable, it is challenging for the residents to live a healthy lifestyle.

According to the Centers for Disease Control and Prevention, *housing availability and quality of housing* refers to the physical condition of the homes in a community, as well as the quality of the social and physical environment where the homes are located. In addition, aspects of housing quality include home safety, space per individual, and the presence of mold, asbestos, or lead. For low-income vulnerable households, there are particular challenges in creating a sense of home in a house that is lacking, which may have substantial effects on health and wellbeing. According to the *American Journal of Public Health*, low-income individuals are twice as likely to occupy homes with severe structural issues, reside in overcrowded homes, and less likely to have proper insulation in their homes. And so, one way in which housing can undermine an individual's health is through *substandard housing*. Substandard housing refers to residential spaces with structural and other physical deficiencies that do not meet health and safety requirements, and thus, endangering the health and safety of the residents that reside within the home. These deficiencies can include exposure to poor indoor air quality, mold, lead, and rodent and cockroach infestations.

Substandard housing can contribute to health conditions such as respiratory conditions, asthma, which is one of the most common chronic diseases among children. Thus, too often low income families are forced to live in substandard housing due to a combination of poverty, lack of affordable housing, and economic instability.

In addition, poor air quality, poor water quality, and exposure to vehicle exhaust emissions, improper waste disposal, and hazardous substances all contribute to compromised health. Certain communities are disproportionately burdened by environmental contamination and health risks.

Economic Security
Economic opportunity motivates and enables individuals to invest in their health; its absence does the exact reverse. Economic Security is defined as having stable, sufficient income that is able to meet one's basic necessities. Economic security is essential for the health and well-being of families. Economic insecurity is defined as an individual residing in a household with income that is below 200 percent of the federal poverty level. An individual's income and socioeconomic status directly affect the quality and quantity of food one can purchase for their family, the quality of housing, the quality of childcare, the ability to prioritize physical activity by joining a gym, ability to pay for clothing, and etc.

The Cost of Living
The United States cost of living today is drastically increasing faster than it has in decades. Unfortunately, average wages for workers are not keeping up with inflation. Thus, this is putting millions of Americans in difficult financial situations. More Americans are being forced to evaluate where they can afford to live and work. As a result, many people are relocating to states that have a lower cost of living in order to save money. Pew Research has stated that approximately 65 percent of low

income adults worry almost everyday about being able to pay their bills. Meanwhile, approximately 57 percent of low income adults say that the price of food and consumer goods significantly affects their household's financial security.

Accessibility to Healthcare

An individual's access to healthcare, including preventive services, can lead to better health outcomes. To understand the ways healthcare impacts the health of a community, it is important to look at conditions such as: employment, income, and education. People who have both health insurance and easy access to care are more likely to receive preventive services such as flu shots, screenings, and vaccines. Preventive services reduce a patient's healthcare spending through early identification of diseases and risk factors. Inadequate health insurance coverage is one of the largest barriers to healthcare access and the unequal distribution of coverage contributes to disparities in health. Out-of-pocket and co-pay costs may contribute to individuals delaying or forgoing the necessary treatment. This includes doctor appointments, annual check-ups/screenings, dental care, and even rationing medication. As reported by the Institute of Medicine United States Committee on Health Insurance, uninsured adults are less likely to receive preventive care. Medical providers must also be equipped with both linguistic and cultural competency, paying attention to issues related to health literacy. The quality of care must be adequate to meet the needs of the patient population. This has important public health implications, and is further explored in Chapter 13.

Transportation
Finally, transportation barriers are often cited as barriers to healthcare access. Transportation issues include, but are not limited to lack of vehicle access, long distances and lengthy travel times to reach health care facilities, transportation costs, inadequate infrastructure, and adverse policies that adversely affect travel. Inconvenient or unreliable transportation can interfere with access to healthcare. It can also lead to rescheduling appointments, delaying treatment, and getting medication. Having access to good transportation options is important for promoting community health.

In Part Three of the book, we will explore each of the Social Determinants of Health and the impact of each factor on patient centered care.

But first, we need to focus on those who influence patient centered care – the providers, the people at the front desk, the administrators managing the hospital department or medical practice, and the healthcare facilities where our treatment is provided. Each influencer has a direct effect on how we, as patients, perceive our care. All that is explored in the next section of the book.

PART TWO
THE INFLUENCERS

Chapter Three

The Providers
By Emelia Behnan, Juhi Patel, Michelle Powell, Yu-Tung (Anna) Lu, and Tasfia Wahid

Introduction
As we will learn in Chapter 20, the patient-provider relationship has a profound impact on the prognosis of a patient and overall outcomes. There is a group of major providers that influence the patient-centered experience. They are directly responsible for creating the relationship and initiating trust with the patient. This chapter will explore the roles and the relationships created by these providers, which includes physicians, dentists, podiatrists, optometrists, chiropractors, nurses, occupational therapists, physical therapists, speech and language pathologists, licensed clinical social workers, psychologists, physician assistants, and pharmacists. The interactions between them as a part of medically diverse team and as individuals with unique approaches are integral to patient-centered care.

Physicians
Physicians are perhaps the most widely recognized providers in the healthcare delivery system. These are the providers who we typically recognize as "our doctors," having earned either the M.D. or D.O. degree after four years of medical school and then further residency training that spans between three and seven years, depending on the specialty. Some doctors have attended an allopathic medical school and earned the M.D. degree, while others have attended an osteopathic medical school and earned the D.O. degree. All physicians have the training and the legal privileges to diagnose, treat, and write prescriptions. Physicians also have one of the greatest impacts on patient-centered care.

There are two broad classes of physicians: primary care and specialists. There are over 135 different specialties in medicine. But it all starts with a primary care physician (PCP). Primary care is a specialty. These doctors have been trained in general medicine, internal medicine, or most often, family medicine. The PCP is recognized as the anchor or facilitator of patient care. Typically, the primary care provider is the first point of contact. They address the "big picture" first, looking at general health as a whole. Most patients visit their PCP at least once a year for a general checkup, and if the patient needs to see a specialist for any diagnosed problem, it is usually the PCP who writes the referral to the specialist, giving the patient the opportunity to make the appointment and the insurance company to pay for the visit with the specialist. One of the major reasons that under most health insurance plans, the patient needs to see the PCP first is to eliminate any unnecessary visits to specialists. The PCP is therefore often considered the gatekeeper of a patient's entry into the healthcare delivery system, deciding when the care of a specialist is really needed, as well as what diagnostic tests the patient will have.

Other Physicians
A patient's complete care also typically includes annual or semi-annual visits to a dentist, as well as perhaps to a podiatrist, an optometrist, or a chiropractor. All of these providers have graduated from their respective schools of training and received a doctoral degree in their discipline. A dentist earns a Doctor of Dental Medicine (DMD) or a Doctor of Dental Surgery (DDS). A podiatrist, who typically treats injuries and issues of the foot and ankle, earns a Doctor of Podiatric Medicine (DPM) and an optometrist, whose practice focuses on the eyes and issues of sight, earns an OD (Doctor of Optometry). A chiropractor, who patients often see for postural problems and body alignment issues, earns a Doctor of Chiropractic (DC). Working both with the primary care

physician as specialists to whom the PCP might refer the patient, many patients, through their healthcare plan, can also have the ability to see these specialists without a referral. In all cases, these doctors are part of an integrated network of providers who together keep the patient healthy, and keep the primary care provider updated on the care the patient receives in their offices. Again, the PCP functions as the anchor, and so, it is important that any medical treatment provided by the other types of doctors is shared with the PCP. This exchange of information between the doctors caring for a patient gives strength to the concept of patient centered care. Likewise, if a patient needs to be treated in an emergency room, and maybe admitted to the hospital, this information is also shared with the PCP so that the doctor has all of the relevant information on the patient. With the advent of electronic medical records, this exchange has become easier, and works to the patient's advantage when the patient sees specialists.

The Role of the Nurse
One of the most important providers in healthcare is the nurse. Most nurses have obtained their RN (Registered Nurse) designation. Some nurses have graduated from a hospital program, while others have an associate's degree from a 2-year college, but most nurses coming into the profession today have earned the Bachelor of Science in Nursing (BSN). The role of the nurse in the healthcare system is fourfold: to monitor the changing condition of the patient, to administer medications and treatments prescribed by an M.D. or D.O., to educate patients about how to manage their illnesses, and to carry out the orders of the doctor in terms of the treatment plan. In terms of patient centered care, it is often said that the nurse and the manner in which he or she attends to the patient either in the hospital or in a medical office can make or break the patient experience, and therefore perhaps is the most important human factor in overall patient centered care. A nurse taking good care of an ill and scared patient with dedication and compassion is priceless. It is important to note

while we are exploring the influence of the providers that a nurse can continue their education to earn an advanced degree, and become a Certified Nurse Practitioner. Because of their rigorous advanced education, the CNP has special legal scope and is allowed by law to diagnose a patient, prescribe medication, and write a treatment plan, just as a physician can. That is why many medical offices and colleges and universities, and even summer camps hire a CNP to be part of their healthcare team, because this type of nurse has the ability to care for a patient at an advanced level.

The Physician Assistant
According to the Tufts University School of Medicine, "physician assistants are integral members of the health care team in many hospitals and clinical practices. The role of the physician assistant (PA) is to practice medicine under the direction and supervision of a licensed physician. Working interdependently with physicians, PA's provide diagnostic and therapeutic patient care in virtually all medical specialties and settings. They take patient histories, perform physical examinations, order laboratory and diagnostic studies, prescribe medications, and develop patient treatment plans. Their job descriptions are as diverse as those of their supervising physicians, and include clinical practice, patient education, team leadership, medical education, health administration, and research." Unlike a CNP, a physician assistant can only diagnose, prescribe, and treat under the direct supervision of a physician. However, like a nurse, the PA is very much a factor in making the patient experience a positive one, and when it comes to patient centered care, the PA is a most important provider, making sure that patient fully understands the diagnosis and the treatment plan, and that the patient consents to the decisions of the medical team. It is interesting to know that most recently, the American Academy of Physician Associates, the professional association to which most PA's belong, has elected to change the name of this profession to *Physician Associates*.

The Pharmacist
In recent years, the pharmacist, who has always been an important member of the healthcare team, has become even more visible to patients, as pharmacists have broadened their scope to be available to administer immunizations and do health consultations with patients. Pharmacists are found both in the retail store as well as behind the scenes working for the online prescription companies. They also play a major role on the hospital team dispensing the medicines that patients require during their hospitalization. The Registered Pharmacist (R.Ph.) of the past is now a Doctor of Pharmacy (Pharm.D) with much broader scope and many more responsibilities. In terms of patient centered care, the pharmacist works closely with prescribing physicians and with patients to make sure that the medicines that are prescribed are compatible with other medications that a patient is taking.

The Allied Health Professions
Finally, we turn our attention to a group of providers who complete the healthcare delivery model. Collectively known as the allied health professions, occupational therapists, physical therapists, speech and language pathologists, licensed clinical social workers, and psychologists are all integral influencers on patient centered care.

The Occupational Therapist
The occupational therapist has a master's degree and earns the credentials of OTR/L, which is a licensed registered occupational therapist. Their main function in medicine is to help people of all ages who have physical, sensory, or cognitive problems. Occupational therapists help with barriers that affect a person's emotional, social, and physical needs. To do this, they use everyday activities, exercises, and other therapies.

The Physical Therapist
The physical therapist today earns a doctorate in physical therapy, which is the DPT degree. The American Physical Therapy Association describes the role of a physical therapist like this: "They help people rehabilitate from devastating injuries, manage chronic conditions, avoid surgery and prescription drugs when possible, and create healthy habits." Additionally, physical therapists treat people across the life span from newborn infants to people nearing the end of their life. They are considered movement specialists. The goal of the activities that they perform is to restore the physical-based functioning and mobility of patients. In doing so, they help to promote a person's well-being and help them enjoy a higher quality of life.

The Speech-Language Pathologist
The speech and language pathologist (SLP) earns a master's degree and according to the American Speech, Language and Hearing Association, speech-language pathologists are experts in communication. SLPs work with people of all ages, from babies to adults, and treat many types of communication and swallowing problems. One of the major patient populations they treat are those with Parkinson's Disease, and often, at the end of life, a speech-language pathologist will be asked to evaluate a patient who can no longer swallow due the progression of the illness, often leading to physicians to consider the intervention of a feeding tube. A related allied professional is the audiologist who specializes in hearing and conditions that result in hearing impairment.

The Mental Health Providers
Finally, there are two other providers. They primarily focus on mental health. The licensed clinical social worker (LCSW) and the psychologist work with the entire medical team to help patients manage trauma and the broad spectrum of mental illnesses. They have a profound influence on patient centered care, as these are the providers who deal with the many emotions of a patient and who help patients accept their medical diagnosis and learn to hopefully cope with it. Dealing with mental illness is as important to the overall health of a patient as dealing with physical illness. Often, the intervention of a LCSW and/or a psychologist can make the difference between a patient having a positive outcome or a negative outcome to their illness. The LSCW has a masters degree in social work with additional training and practical hours completed. The psychologist earns a Doctor of Psychology degree or Psy.D. and is involved in what has become known as talk therapy to help a patient through trauma, depression, and other mental health challenges.

The Influence of Providers on Patient Centered Care
All of the providers explored in this chapter indeed influence patient centered care. To most providers, patient centered care is a priority of their practice of medicine, and most providers recognize that the way they treat and relate to a patient can enhance the patient experience or greatly compromise the patient experience. It is often said that patient centered care begins with and ends with the provider, but in the next chapter, we are going to look at another major influence, the support staff, the folks who work behind the front desk and those who have a more clinical role and assist with taking vital signs and welcoming the patient before the patient is seen by the healthcare provider.

Chapter Four

The Support Staff
By Abigail Arient

The support staff of healthcare facilities play a very important part in the entire process and system of healthcare. These folks are often both the first and last people seen by the patient during any sort of visit to a healthcare facility. And therefore, these team members play a large part in patient centered care. This chapter will explore the role that the support staff plays and how patient and support staff interactions may vary, and will also address common concerns and complaints of patients regarding the support staff.

The Two Major Types of Support Staff

Administrative Support Staff
These are the people who both directly and indirectly support the provider. The positions of support staff include the practice or department administrators, the front desk staff, and the billing staff.

Clinical Support Staff
These are the people who have roles that are more patient focused and hands on, such as medical assistants, ultrasound and imaging technicians, dental hygienists in a dental practice, EKG technicians in a cardiology practice, phlebotomists, and other lab or sample collecting technicians.

The Essential Roles of the Support Staff

Without the support staff, healthcare would not be the same. Their various roles both directly and indirectly assist the practitioner in the operation of their office or clinic. Often the background heroes, these essential staff members are the folks who keep offices and clinics functional. It takes a team working together in order to provide proper patient care, and without the support staff, the base of the pyramid would not exist and the team would crumble. Customer service skills are not only needed when face to face with patients but also over the phone as well. With many different hats to wear and various tasks to juggle throughout the day, the support staff is the backbone of a practice or office.

How Common Patient Complaints and Concerns Affect Patient Centered Care

Dealing with the more tertiary parts of healthcare such as medical billing, the support staff is also very involved with the business side of healthcare. Many offices also outsource their billing through separate companies as office staff may not have billing experience and in-house billers can create unnecessary costs. It is important to address the complaints by patients about the support staff. According to Becker's Hospital Review, a major barometer of patient satisfaction throughout the United States, the patient's number one complaint regarding their time and experience at their doctor's office is how the front desk staff treats the patient. The front desk staff is often criticized for being rude, harsh, and unprofessional with their customer service. While some of these complaints are warranted and true, it does not change the fact that at the end of the day. the support staff often takes the brunt of patient complaints, concerns, and frustrations.

As far as the complaints towards the more clinically involved support staff, these grievances are often focused on a lack of proper bedside manner. Nurses and medical assistants can sometimes be seen as cold or grumpy. Other clinical support staff such as nurse practitioners or physician assistants can feel looked down upon as they are not "real" doctors, but other members of the healthcare team who help support the doctor.

It is important to note that just as there are many complaints from the patients, one must also recognize that the front staff also have complaints of their own about the patients. Unless these concerns are resolved at both ends of the relationship, the patient experience is compromised. The folks at the front desk often feel overwhelmed and burned out. This sentiment is shared by clinical and non-clinical support staff alike. Often stretched far too thin, especially in times when there are many healthcare concerns by patients, such as what healthcare offices and facilities faced with the COVID-19 pandemic, healthcare workers everywhere are tired and this includes the front desk staff. While many people had the luxury to change to working remotely at home at the onset of the pandemic, healthcare workers did not have such luxury, and instead, because they were deemed essential workers, these folks were on the front lines, at risk everyday, in order to maintain the healthcare system, allowing doctors to still see patients. This overall feeling of exhaustion and burnout is one that has driven many to search for alternate career opportunities. While many patient concerns regarding the support staff are valid, it is also important to take a step back to acknowledge and appreciate all that the support staff have to deal with.

Resolving the Conflicts for the Sake of Better Patient Centered Care

As the term suggests, patient centered care places the patient first and aims to do this in many different ways. One major way is through patient advocacy. Patient advocacy can be done by addressing valid complaints made regarding the front desk and other support staff. It can also be provided by having a system where a patient feels that they are heard in their concerns and other issues. where an environment exists based on trust and understanding. While patient centered care approaches are important and do need to be implemented, patients also need to try to mutually respect and understand the support staff. If both patient and support staff can approach one another from this mutual respect perspective, one of patience, empathy, and understanding, then common complaints and concerns can be cleared up and resolved.

Consider this. When you call a hospital or medical practice, the person at the other end of the call is most probably a member of the support staff. At the moment you call, they may be involved in many other things at the same time, and so, it is important for the patient to show compassion and understanding just as you want them to show you the same. Stay patient with the folks at the front desk. Be sure to thank them for working with you. Understand that they are under constant pressure to do the best job possible for the many patients they encounter each day. Be mindful that they want to help you, but we, as patients, need to try to help them do their job, as well. We need to have the information they require when we call or when we visit a practice, we need to comply with the signing of paperwork, even if it sometimes seems unnecessary, and we need to be patient with them if they cannot answer a question quickly, especially when they are obligated to have the provider answer it.

The support staff has a major responsibility to be the bridge between the providers and the patients, and to help make a visit a good experience for every patient.

Chapter Five

The Administrators
By Mason La Fleur

Administrators, like support staff, not only share the responsibility of providing top-notch quality healthcare but also creating an enjoyable and rewarding work environment for their employees. They oversee all that goes on in their organization, making decisions that are in the best interest of their patients and their staff. And there are several occurrences where both of their needs are contradictory to each other. Patients are looking to the administrators to provide them with high-quality care, around the clock service, and in some cases, for the administrators to make life-saving decisions.

Healthcare administrators direct and make crucial business decisions for the healthcare organization. Without healthcare administrators, the healthcare industry as a whole would collapse because these men and women manage the business of healthcare. Like many other industries, healthcare has a hierarchy of departments, and it is important for the patient to understand how a typical healthcare facility is structured and the way the facility is managed. It is even more important that the patient know to whom to turn when there is an issue with the patient's care.

The Education of a Healthcare Administrator
Most healthcare administrators have a Masters in Health Administration (MHA), a Masters in Business Administration (MBA), or a Masters in Public Health (MPH). With these degrees, some also need various certifications depending on which state they reside in, and also what kind of healthcare

organization they are leading. There are also administrators who have earned a bachelors degree in Healthcare Administration from a school of business, which prepares them to enter the profession and serve in an administrative role earlier in their career because they have a complete background in both healthcare administration and business. At the same time, most healthcare organizations, especially bigger hospitals that are university-affiliated, have administrator in training (AIT) programs that allow recent college graduates to pursue a master's degree while working for the healthcare organization. The hospital pays for the classes for the AIT student, in exchange for a commitment to work for the hospital for an agreed-upon amount of time, after the degree has been completed.

With their leadership, collaboration, and problem-solving abilities, healthcare administrators are positioned to lead in all types of healthcare facilities. They can manage hospitals, outpatient clinics and medical offices, long-term care facilities, clinical labs, and hospices. Their duties may differ based on the type of healthcare facility they manage. However, their general responsibilities remain largely the same. In a hospital, administrators collaborate with a team of leaders who oversee the daily operations of each department. In this setting, they review budgets, write new policies, and appoint new medical staff. Outpatient care facility administrators play a senior-level role to meet the needs of patients with high-quality ambulatory care services. Outpatient care refers to patient treatments that are completed during the daytime without overnight stays. These types of facilities include urgent care centers, one-day surgery, primary care and specialty medical practices, mental health facilities, rehab therapy practices, diagnostic imaging centers, chemotherapy, drug rehabilitation, or dialysis. Clinical laboratory administrators oversee a medical testing facility and manage all operations such as overseeing test procedures; analyzing requests for tests and equipment; and assisting with budgets. Clinical laboratory administrators can work in private and government labs, doctor's offices, hospitals, and clinics. They may be trained to deal with infectious or hazardous materials and are typically required to wear protective gear when handling such materials. A hospice administrator manages an end-of-life care facility. Hospices are dedicated to supporting the emotional, physical, and social needs of patients and their families.

Despite not having regular direct contact with patients, administrators make decisions that significantly impact the experiences of patients. They must adhere to the patient-centered model of care - an approach in which a patient's specific health needs and preferences drive all health care decisions. Administrators can encourage a more positive care environment for patients and employees alike while also ensuring their healthcare organization establishes patient-centric goals that focus on the Social Determinants of Health.

One main focus that healthcare administrators have to deal with is making sure that their practice complies with government regulations, which includes laws and polices at the federal, state, and local levels. Healthcare as a whole has been regulated for over 150 years, and has been described by some administrators as, "A maze with no end in sight". Some government agencies that are heavily involved in healthcare regulation include the **Centers for Disease Control and Prevention (CDC)**, the **World Health Organization (WHO)**, and the **Food and Drug Administration (FDA)**. They do things like conduct health and safety inspections, investigate epidemics and pandemics, oversee public health, test and approve medicine, and make policy about healthcare practices. This is what most people think of when they hear healthcare regulation. Healthcare administrators have to constantly make sure that their buildings, staff, and other assets are complying with this complex system that has been put in place.

While it's important for administrators to make sure their healthcare facilities are within the legal requirements of operation, it's equally important for them to make decisions that help build their facilities and generate revenue for their business. This means that they need to be able to have an extensive knowledge of business, or employ people who do, in order to keep the healthcare facility financially solvent. This involves attracting patients, expanding to different geographic locations, seeking out different demographics, and training staff to expand their treatment options. Improvement of the business side of healthcare usually happens behind the scenes, and most patients and their loved ones may not even realize it's happening. Often, when a healthcare organization announces a new state-of-the-art building, new technology, or begins to offer a new service, there have been weeks, months, or even years of preparation and planning that go into that announcement.

How Administrators Impact Patient Centered Care
Patient centered care is a topic that we've been focusing on throughout this book, and now we're going to look at it through the eyes of the healthcare administrator, and how the decisions they make impact patient centered care.

One main focus that healthcare administrators have regarding patient centered care is the mission, vision, and values of their healthcare facility. Each healthcare facility has a mission statement, and the best mission statements describe the goals of the healthcare facility, and the process that must be in place to achieve those goals. Spectrum Health is a major healthcare corporation located in Grand Rapids, Michigan, where they own and operate multiple hospitals, outpatient clinics, ambulatory care centers, and other healthcare facilities. Their mission is as follows: "Improve health, instill humility, and inspire hope." Their mission statement is very short, concise, and gets their point across in as little words as possible. This message provides their patients with an idea of what it is that Spectrum Health is trying to achieve and gives each patient peace of mind when being cared for by Spectrum.

At the same time, Spectrum Health also does a great job at clarifying their values. Their vision states, "A future where health is simple, affordable, equitable, and exceptional."

They use a simple, one sentence message that is effective and easy to understand. Spectrum Health is trying to communicate with their patients about what they want the future to hold for their company, and then goes into greater detail about the steps they are taking in order to make that happen. It is messages like these that reassure the patients who choose Spectrum Health that they are in good hands, and that the care that's being provided to them is centered to only them specifically.

Implementing Patient Centered Care
Administrators are also tasked with the responsibility of all direct-care staff in their healthcare facility, and it's important to be able to make sure everyone knows what their roles are, and how they fit into the bigger picture. In order for patient centered care to be successful, staff members need to be fully committed to their work, and should take pride in the work that they do, not only as individuals, but also as an organization. It's equally as important for employees to understand the work of other staff members, and where their responsibility ends. A front desk receptionist needs to be able to coordinate with the patient transport staff, and that transport staff needs to work with nurses, and those nurses need to be able to work with technicians, and so on. It's very common in healthcare workplaces for staff to blame other areas of the facility when someone has made a mistake, saying things like "I wasn't responsible for that" or "That falls under their responsibility" and this mindset goes back and forth between different departments. In order to break that cycle of "passing the buck", it's important for departments that work together often to understand each other's roles in detail, and coordinate where one staff member's responsibility ends and another one starts.

In a healthcare setting, it's always better to over-communicate than to be left in the dark. Shifting this mindset will not only increase productivity, but it will make staff better at their job and directly impact the patient's experience in a positive way.

Administrators need to also work hand in hand with *patient advocates*. Patient advocates spend most of their day listening to patient concerns, so they are able to get a great understanding of what a healthcare facility is doing right, and what they're doing wrong. Working with patient advocates can help an administrative team gain insight to what may be slipping through the cracks, and then implement change into their facility in order to better the patient's overall experience.

In healthcare facilities in which I have personally worked, there have been instances when independent patient advocates come in and survey patients and staff. This allows for the administration to know what needs to be changed to meet the expectations of their patients, and for their staff members as well. Patient surveys and staff surveys are anonymous, which allow patients and staff to respond freely about the facility and their employer. It may be tough for administrators to hear what their patients or staff members have to say, but in order to make change for the better, administrators need to put those voices first.

Finding the Right Administrator When You Need One
In a typical hospital or other large healthcare facility, there are clinical departments and there are support departments. Each department has a main department administrator. As an example, in the area of support departments, one might need to reach the head administrator of the operations, financial affairs, legal, human resources, housekeeping, facilities management, medical records, or the environmental services department. In the area of clinical departments, the patient may need to reach out to the head administrator of a medical

department such as the emergency room, the departments of surgery or maternity or intensive care, pediatrics, or diagnostic imaging. There are usually over 350 different departments in a hospital, and there could be over 10 different departments in a large medical practice. For each major department in a facility, there are directors and managers who oversee the administration of divisions of the department such as the billing department under financial affairs, or the collection department, also under financial affairs. Directors and managers of divisions are also found on the clinical side of the operation such as under the Department of Medicine, you would find a different administrator for each division such as an administrator for general medicine, one for endocrinology, another one for cardiology, or ENT, or pulmonology, or pediatrics. While administrators don't see patients on a regular basis, patients can meet with them if needed and they greatly influence how the healthcare organization is operated, the quality of care patients receive, and the level of patient centered care that is delivered.

The next chapter explores how healthcare facilities - their size, their structure, their purpose - have an impact on patient centered care.

Chapter Six

The Healthcare Facilities
By Mason La Fleur

This chapter focuses on the role that different healthcare facilities play when looking at patient centered care, and how each healthcare facility differs from another. While each facility shares a common goal of making people healthy and happy, the way that each facility does that can be expressed in many ways.

Hospitals, nursing homes, ambulatory care centers, and urgent care centers are just some of the facilities that we think of when you think about healthcare. These facilities welcome people who are ill or hurting with open arms with the goal of making them feel better again, and they do so without question. With pain and sickness, there is vulnerability that comes with it. Patients expect their providers to give them the best possible care and treatment during their stay at a facility, but that can look different with each facility.

However, in order to dive deep into how each facility operates, we first need to define some terms.

AMBULATORY CARE CENTERS: As I explained in the previous chapter, ambulatory care, otherwise known as outpatient care, is care provided to patients without admitting them to a longer term care facility. Ambulatory care facilities can include (but not be limited to), urgent care centers, family practices, specialty practices, and hospital outpatient centers.

NURSING HOMES: A nursing home is a place for people who don't need to be cared for in a hospital but cannot be cared for at home. Typically these people are elderly, many of whom require 24 hour care.

ASSISTED LIVING CARE CENTERS: Assisted living care centers are very similar to nursing homes, however the patients that live in assisted living care centers usually require more intensive care than those that live in nursing homes. This could be anything from memory care to mobility care. Assisted living care centers also have more specialized staff that are experienced in geriatric care. At the same time, many retirement communities that an older person may move to after selling their home or apartment, provide independent living for those who are still able to enjoy living with independence including driving themselves, shopping for themselves, traveling, and taking advantage of the social activities of the retirement community. However, these retirement communities also offer assisted living care in the event that the independent resident later requires medical assistance or round-the-clock care.

HOSPICE CARE FACILITIES: These are healthcare facilities that specialize in making their patients as comfortable as possible at the end of life. Once the patient has come to terms with death, very specialized healthcare professionals make the patient comfortable and peaceful in their final days. Decisions for the patient can also be made by loved ones or family members if the patient cannot make decisions for themselves, and the hospice nurses also provide comfort and support to the families, as well.

BURNOUT: As we learned in the account by physical therapist Dr. Logan Nester in the earlier section on Providers, burnout is the emotional, mental, and physical exhaustion caused from working at too fast a pace, working too long, or doing too much. Burnout has been on the rise in healthcare workers in recent years due to the COVID-19 pandemic, with staff shortages and extremely stressful work environments. The word burnout is interesting because that is literally what is happening on the cellular level; the cells are burning themselves to death.

EMR: EMR, or electronic medical records, are a digital version of a traditional paper-based medical record for a patient. EMR's can include basic vitals, treatment plan, medication prescriptions, special notes, and whatever else a healthcare professional needs to know when going to treat a patient. EMR is becoming more popular as technology progresses, and many healthcare facilities have made the switch from paper to digital, or are in the process of doing so. The great value of the EMR system is that a patient's medical history and current treatment can be shared with any doctor treating the patient.

The Reasonable Expectations of a Patient in a Facility

Every time a patient walks into a healthcare facility, they should be able to have a general idea of what's to come in terms of their care. Whether it is a hospital, nursing home, assisted living center, hospice care, urgent care, or other type of facility, every patient has expectations of how they want to be treated and the kind of care they want to receive. Patients expect to be treated with kindness and respect, while receiving the best care possible from the people who are there to care for them. However, this can look drastically different depending on the type of healthcare facility.

The Hospital
The main goal a hospital is to get you feeling better and transition you into ambulatory care services as quickly as possible. If a patient is admitted into the hospital for a broken leg, for example, they would most likely have to undergo surgery to repair the bone, and be put into a cast, and leave the

hospital with crutches or a wheelchair. Once the patient has been discharged and the patient has recovered from the initial surgery, the patient would be referred to a physical therapist so that they can continue the recovery process from home, making that hospital bed available for the next patient. If there was an infection, however, or other complications down the road of recovery, the hospital would readmit the patient once again until the healthcare professionals had resolved that complication. Hospitals, while their focus is the practice of medicine, they are also a business. Hospitals always want to have beds available for incoming patients, and so, their goal is to keep patients moving throughout the recovery process as efficiently as possible, and without compromising the health of a patient, hospitals try to discharge patients as soon as medically reasonable. One of the major problems with this goal is that often patients are sent home too early and become sick again, creating a need for the patient to be readmitted to the facility.

Long-Term Care Facilities
Nursing homes and assisted living centers are operated much differently than hospitals. At their core, they are very similar in the sense that they want to make their patients feel better, and they are also businesses at the end of the day. However, these healthcare facilities are much more focused on patient relationships. The average length of stay in a hospital is four and a half days, and during that time, the patient sees several different staff members whose job is to take care of them. Long term care facilities like nursing homes and assisted living care centers are much more focused on things like bedside manners and patient-caretaker relationships because their patients interact with the same staff every single day. Long term care facilities also have to have a bigger budget for things like dining services, custodial services, maintenance services, and grounds crew. All of these extra accommodations are used as selling points to patients and their loved ones when the long term care facility talks to patients and their families about choosing the facility.

Ambulatory Care Facilities

Ambulatory care services, on the other hand, are focused on how to find the perfect balance between quality of care, and the number of patients their individual facility can take in. Ambulatory care services, as stated above, are healthcare services that are usually made by appointment, and each visit lasts a couple of hours on average. Ambulatory care is an umbrella term used in healthcare, and practices such as family doctors, dentists, physical therapists, specialists, urgent care centers, ambulatory surgical centers, and dialysis clinics fall into this category of facilities. These types of healthcare facilities are working to provide their patients with high quality care, while also trying to maximize the number of patients they can see on a daily basis. In addition, if a patient is visiting an ambulatory care service, they are most likely doing so in a non-emergent context. There are a few outliers of course, one example of that being a visit to the dentist for a broken tooth.

Ambulatory care accounts for about 65% of all care in the United States, according to McKinsey and Company, a private healthcare research organization. This number continues to rise with more and more people taking advantage of the convenience of urgent care centers in their area.

Patient Expectations

A recent study explored how patients perceive their healthcare experience across a range of different health care facilities. The researchers studied different patients with various degrees of illness and injuries, and in various different healthcare settings. They conducted interviews with these patients, asking them questions about their demographics, basic medical history, their experience so far and expectations of what was to come while staying at their particular healthcare facility. To no surprise, the most important patient expectation was that the patient would have an improvement of overall health. Interestingly, another aspect of healthcare that was consistently found in studies of different patients was the acceptance of the limitations of individual healthcare workers. Many patients who required extra care understood that the nurses, doctors, and other direct care staff who cared for them could only do so much as individuals, which shifted the patients blame to the healthcare organization as a whole. Quotes were taken from different patients saying things like "They're doing the best they can." and, "The doctors are very good, but the health system is not". Some of the patients did expect more from the individual healthcare workers, citing that some of them were rude, had poor bedside manner, and did not communicate things in a way that the patient could understand. This highlights that there are aspects of patient care that may not be taken as seriously by healthcare professionals, but mean a lot to individual patients, especially those that want to understand what's going on with their bodies and be involved in decision making of their own personal care.

This study did a very good job at looking across the healthcare spectrum as a whole, interviewing patients who stayed in different healthcare facilities, had varying severity of injury/illness, and patients with different demographics. The results reflect patient expectations of not only hospitals, but also nursing homes, outpatient clinics, assisted living centers, and urgent care centers.

Are Healthcare Facilities Meeting Patient Expectations?

Patient centered care can take shape in many different ways across the different types of healthcare facilities. However, there are common themes among each of these facilities surrounding patient centered care. These include shared decision making, customized care, and information sharing. Shared decision making is exactly how it sounds, allowing for patients and their family members to come to a shared conclusion with a health professional on how to proceed with their health. This allows for the patient and their loved ones to feel more involved in their own healthcare, and communicates to them that their opinion is valued, which can improve their overall experience.

For example, if someone comes into the hospital needing to be treated for chest pain, and it is not an emergency situation and options can be discussed, there are multiple different courses of treatment the doctor may recommend for this patient. If the doctor or other healthcare professional chooses to do so, they can administer treatment without asking the patient what their personal opinion is on it, and without discussing it with the patient's family members or loved ones. While that may be the most effective treatment plan for that patient, the healthcare professional is leaving everyone in the dark when they should be able to come to a shared conclusion on how to move forward. If the healthcare professional were to discuss the different treatment options with the patient, and let them bring their past experiences with their personal health to the table, the patient's overall experience would be better and there may be a more effective treatment plan administered.

For a healthcare facility, allowing patients to be able to make informed decisions about their care is a key component to patient satisfaction. This idea also overlaps with customized care, and making sure the staff in each healthcare facility knows that their patients are not going to react exactly the way the textbooks say they should. This is true especially in long - term care facilities, where the focus on building good patient-caretaker relationships is much more valued. If a caretaker is able to recognize patterns about their patients, noticing even the little things, it makes a bigger impact on those patients than most believe. Simple things like leaving a glass of water on their bedside stand if you know a patient wakes up thirsty, or giving a patient a stack of magazines because you know how much they love to read can go a long way in building a positive relationship with that patient.

Effect of Physical Environments
These patient centered practices look different with each healthcare facility, which is why it's important for these facilities to be constantly evolving to make sure that their patients are at the center of the facility's operation. A study done by the National Library of Medicine looked at how the physical environment of a facility can also have an impact on how patients feel when they are a patient at a healthcare facility. These features can be simple, like having calm, soothing music playing in a waiting room, or making the paint on the walls a neutral color. It can also bring much harder challenges, like having a strong information technology sector that provides constant communication lines between the patient and the caretaker. Healthcare facilities are built around what the patient experiences, and facilities try to eliminate the barriers to the patient experience. This is why there are always so many signs in hospitals telling patients and family members where things are located, how to get there, and where they currently are in relation to things like the cafeteria and the parking lots.

Healthcare facilities are built to serve their patients in the best way they know how, and with the constant progress in technology they are able to improve the care that is given to their patients, as well as the communication they can provide to the patients' loved ones. As we learned from hospital executive Beth Duffy earlier in the book, when you look at healthcare facilities through a broader lens, every decision that is made during the building process is made with a patient's need in mind. There are some aspects of healthcare facilities that are so subtle, that can go unnoticed by a patient, but are important and can positively impact a patient's stay. Most of the time the patient does not even realize it. So the next time you go into a hospital, nursing home, urgent care, or other type of healthcare facility, try and notice some of the smaller details that might make your stay there a little bit better.

PART THREE
THE INFLUENCES

Chapter Seven

The Impact of a Patient's Education

By Julianna Celestin, Abigail Arient, and Anooshka Shukla

Basic education is an integral part of being healthy. Education gives people the tools they need to lead fulfilling lives, thrive personally, and contribute to their communities. In addition, education makes it more likely for a person to access quality healthcare, find employment that pays a living wage and hopefully provides health insurance, and live in a shapeless, non-polluted environment. Education teaches a person to use their mind: learning, thinking, solving problems, to keep the body in shape. Educated patients are more able to comprehend their health needs. For instance, an individual with a college degree may have better skills to evaluate conflicting or complex information they are told by a doctor. Meanwhile, an individual with less formal education may be less prepared to decide between reliable and unreliable information, in addition to following directions, adequately advocating for themselves and their families, and communicating effectively with healthcare professionals.

What are Adverse Childhood Experiences?
Adverse Childhood Experiences are potential experiences a child may endure that can cause stress, potentially leading to trauma. Research conducted by the Centers for Disease Control and Prevention cites that toxic stress from adverse childhood experiences can alter brain development and affect the body's response to stress. It continues to elaborate that adverse childhood experiences are linked to chronic health

problems, mental illness, and substance misuse in adulthood. Brain development is a continuous process throughout life that goes through sensitive periods during which stressors and nurturing experiences can have everlasting effects.

Effect of Adverse Childhood Experiences on Health
Education can be linked to health by exposure to conditions, beginning in early childhood, which can affect both education and health. It is the ordinary day-to-day experiences in family, neighborhood, school, and work dynamics that affect the brain and body functions and promote those health-damaging behaviors. Adverse effects of stress on the developing brain and behavior are significant. It can affect performance in school and explain learning setbacks. As a result, children exposed to stress may also be drawn to risky behaviors. High-risk behaviors can be described as behaviors that increase the risk of disease and [or] injury, which could potentially result in disability, death, and [or] social problems. The most common high-risk behaviors include violence, alcoholism, tobacco use, risky sexual behaviors, and eating disorders. Thus, resulting in poor health. Poor health can cause education setbacks starting at a young age. For instance, children with chronic illnesses such as asthma and other chronic illnesses may experience recurrent absences and difficulty concentrating in classes. Children who grow up in low-income and [or] elevated stressed environments or neighborhoods face a double burden; their living conditions might disturb and disrupt their education.

Education should be recognized as an essential requirement for the disruption of the cycle of poverty and inequalities in health. Some evidence provided by the Center for Educational Research and Innovation of The Organization for Economic Co-operation and Development (OECD) suggested that education is strongly linked to health determinants such as preventive care. According to the *Annual Review of Public Health*, education improves health because it increases effective agency, enhancing a sense of personal control that encourages and enables a healthy lifestyle. In addition, education exposes individuals to a wealth of information that might prompt them to make healthier decisions, one of them being access to healthcare services. Education offers opportunities to learn more about health and health risks, both in the form of health education in the school curriculum and by giving individuals the health literacy to draw on, later in life, and absorb messages about important lifestyle choices to prevent or manage diseases. A clear understanding of the health benefits of education can therefore serve as the key to reducing health disparities and improving the well-being of future populations.

Impact of Health Literacy on Patient Centered Care
According to the Health Resources and Services Administration, health literacy is defined as the degree to which individuals can obtain, process, and understand basic health information needed to make appropriate health decisions. Low health literacy is more prevalent in older adults, minority populations, those who have low socioeconomic status, and medically underserved people.

Educational access directly impacts patient-centered care. Previous studies have found that a patient's level of education was directly connected to their satisfaction and understanding of healthcare. For a majority of adults in America, education is a big factor in their lack of health literacy. Those with lower health literacy should not be held in a position of fault as their situation could be the result of many factors working against them. Similarly, patients with high health literacy should not receive preferential treatment for their greater schema and literacy surrounding health and wellness. As such this brings up the importance of individualizing patient-centered care and patient education and resulting health literacy are prime examples of how such social determinants of health can vary across populations.

Impact of Health Literacy on Navigating the Health System

Limited health literacy and limited general literacy can prevent people from learning about health, using medication properly, and taking advantage of preventative services. Patients who are unable to understand their providers are more prone to not following medication directions, the effects of their health diagnoses, seeking health care, knowing the differences between risky and healthy behaviors, properly documenting their health history, and managing their health conditions. Health literacy significantly allows patients to take control of their well-being by making intelligent healthcare choices, improving their communication with their healthcare providers, and equipping them with the vital information necessary to advocate for themselves in a medical setting.

Educational Access and Patient Health Outcomes and Trends

As much as doctors and support staff try their best to explain everything in a way that the patient can understand, at times there are misunderstandings between these parties. These misunderstandings in part are due to the varying levels of education of the parties involved. An expert in the field of medicine, the doctor or practitioner is a highly educated individual whereas the patient's education level drastically varies. For example, if a patient is unsure of proper dosing and how to take a prescribed medication from their doctor and unknowingly misuses the medication, this can result in health complications. The level of education can greatly impact one's access to quality care as someone's level of education impacts job opportunities. For example, according to the *Quarterly Journal of Economics*, someone with a college degree is more likely to make more than their counterparts who do not have a degree and be eligible for jobs that have higher compensation and benefits packages. These benefit packages can impact someone's access to healthcare based on insurance eligibility and coverage. Therefore, access to quality and affordable care covered by insurance is related to a patient's level of education. In a sense, this can discriminate against patients of lower levels of education who lack the same access and opportunities as more educated patients have, in terms of health insurance and other benefits that can come with jobs that require higher levels of education. While public aid programs such as Medicaid do aim to help ease that gap in healthcare faced by low-income patients, it highlights the fact that without such programs, access to care would be non-existent for some patients.

Bridging the Gap Using Cultural Competency

Cultural competency is one of the main ingredients in decreasing the disparities within the healthcare system among various racial and ethnic groups. The increasing population growth of racial and ethnic communities presents a challenge to the healthcare delivery service in the states. A 2019 study published in the JAMA Network Open, noted that data collected from approximately 5.4 million individuals showed a lack of progress in eliminating health inequities across the country.

Effective communication skills are an important skill. Communication has always been a vital component of healthcare service and a fundamental way to improve quality care. Physicians must promote patient education and engagement through improvement in patients' health literacy. As described in the previous section, health literacy is defined as the capacity to seek, understand, and act on health information. Data has shown that many healthcare providers do not utilize and converse with vocabulary and [or] terminology patients understand. Medical care is full of jargon, which most patients are not familiar with. Additionally, in relation to being culturally competent, effective communication is key. The appropriate utilization of jargon that the patient can easily understand can help with the communication. The appropriate utilization of interpreters can also help. The Patient Bill of Rights states that if a patient does not speak English, the patient is entitled to request an interpreter during a healthcare encounter. Health interpreters can help healthcare providers to understand the patient's symptoms and what diagnostic tests should be run. Language and communication barriers can affect the amount and quality of health care the patient receives.

Telehealth: Bridging the Gap Using Technology
Telehealth and other technologies can make it easier for patients to access care services and health records. Improving this type of access can help improve the quality of care for hard-to-reach patients. Advancements in technology and digital platforms have made it extremely easy to access all kinds of resources with a touch of a screen, including the opportunity to meet with a physician or other healthcare professional without having to set foot in a healthcare facility. By definition according to the Centers for Disease Control and Prevention, telemedicine is the utilization of electronic information and telecommunication technology to get healthcare services. The patient needs to utilize a device such as a phone or a laptop with an internet connection. Telemedicine includes phone calls, video chats, emails, and text messages.

Telemedicine allows healthcare professionals to evaluate, diagnose, and treat patients at a distance utilizing telecommunications. The approach has been through a striking evolution in the last decade due to the internet, and it is becoming an increasingly important part of the American healthcare infrastructure. By utilizing telemedicine, patients no longer are required to wait in waiting rooms for hours to get medical attention. Using patient portals set up by hospitals and medical practices, patients can book appointments remotely and contact doctors as quickly as possible. Telemedicine provides patients and healthcare providers the same face-to-face engagement that would be done if it was in person. Furthermore, telemedicine cuts transportation costs and time they would have missed from being away from work.

In order to improve the overall health status of the United States, the many barriers that center around education can be reduced through various options and methods. One option is the creation of additional schooling such as vocational training, alternate schools, socio-emotionally skill training, and counseling to help increase the rate of graduation. With these implementations, there is an increase from the baseline rate of 84.1% to 85.8%, which is closer to the goal of 90.7%. Related are programs that increase the betterment of math skills. A popular ongoing study called *Healthy People 2030* states that those who do significantly well in math tend to experience better health outcomes.

Additionally, certain programs pertaining to certain public health topics can influence the overall health status outcome. Healthy People 2030 states that implementing a program that revolves around safer sexual health education as well as overall understanding of reproductive health can lead to an increase in using birth control, reducing pregnancies, and lowering the STI rates in that age group, which leads to better health outcomes.

With these objectives, goals, and supplemental programs in mind, the barriers preventing the reduction in health disparities due to education levels can be implemented and addressed. But there is still progress to be made. Education indeed has a significant impact on the patient experience.

Chapter Eight

The Impact of a Patient's Gender
By Anat Ferleger

This chapter will focus on how the identified gender of a patient impacts their perception of patient centered care. Utilizing the medical sociology approach and using the Social Determinants of Health as the basis, the chapter will examine how the identified gender of a patient can impact their role as a patient and their interaction with providers and facilities.

The Basic Inequities of Access to Healthcare – Men and Women
Men tend to utilize the healthcare system far less than women. Many factors are likely to play a role in this. For one, there are gaps within health insurance that leave men unable to receive the same benefits and preventative care as women. Toxic masculinity, patriarchal views, cultural values and societal norms also likely play a role.

According to the World Health Organization, what is known as *the "toxic masculinity" mindset* is likely a primary causative factor for health disparities between men and women. Men tend to put themselves at greater risk for injury and illness and are less willing to ask for help than women. This mindset not only increases their risk for physical illness or injury, but also increases one's risk for suicide. According to the American Foundation for Suicide Prevention, men are four times as likely to commit suicide as women. It is evident that "toxic masculinity" norms play a role in shaping men's expectations and behaviors, directly impacting their health. Brown University, as well as other scattered universities around the country are creating open, safe spaces for students, young and old, to unpack and unlearn toxic masculinity norms. Expanding programs with similar missions is one way to help lead the way in reversing this toxic mindset for future generations.

Equity is another large issue when it comes to men's healthcare in our country. The Affordable Care Act lacks coverage for basic male healthcare needs, while many packages are specifically tailored for women. This compromises the incentive for men to purchase healthcare insurance. Under the ACA, a comprehensive annual well-women visit is covered at no cost. This includes a full checkup, separate from any sickness or injury visit. The visit focuses on "preventative care for women" and includes immunizations, patient education, diet and exercise counseling, as well as mental health screenings. While men are far more likely to live an unhealthy lifestyle, and have a shorter lifespan than women, there are no comparable visits for those who identify as male. This leaves men to take their health into their own hands and advocate for their own care, which most do not do.

A study conducted by the Commonwealth Fund confirmed that this is a large issue within our country. It found that a majority of men in America do not receive basic medical care, such as routine checkups and counseling. The percentage of men who ignore symptoms of illness or injury is on the rise. Three times as many men as women have not seen any type of physician within the last year. More than half the men surveyed have not had a physical exam, or had blood work done in the previous year. 60% of men 50 and older have not been screened for colon cancer, and 41% have not being screened for prostate cancer. One in four men say they would wait as long as possible before receiving medical care after a concerning issue presents itself.

Providing equity would not only give men an incentive to buy insurance, but it would remove gender-based discriminations giving men the same chance at living long and healthy lives.

Women Access the Healthcare System More Than Men

Studies have found that women typically spend far more on healthcare throughout their lifetime than men. This is possibly related to longevity. The lifespan of a woman in the United States is 81 years, while the average man's life expectancy is 76.1. While this does give women an extra five years to acquire medical bills, this is likely not to be the main factor in why women utilize healthcare more frequently than men. A study by The National Center for Health Statistics found that between the year 1995 and 2011, women made 30% more visits to physicians than men. Women tend to seek preventative care more frequently than men, and as they begin to have children, the number of visits increases dramatically.

What is Gender Bias?

Gender bias is a global issue. In 2020, a United Nations report found that up to 90% of people have a gender bias against women. Gender bias refers to a type of prejudice that favors one gender of another. In more cases than not, these biases favor men. Many are not aware of their own biases. *Explicit biases* are those that one is aware of, while *implicit biases* are unconscious. Both types of bias influence one's behavior. While this report stems across all fields, it plays a vital role in why biases exist in the healthcare setting.

Gender Bias Against Women in Healthcare

According to a survey done by *TODAY*, more than half of women believe that gender discrimination in the healthcare setting is a serious issue compared to one third of men. One in five women has reported that they felt like their symptoms were dismissed in a healthcare setting. 17% of women say that they feel as though they are treated differently in healthcare settings compared to only 6% of men.

It has been shown that the perception women have about the gender bias that exists in healthcare is correct. Women who present with the same symptoms and conditions as men do not receive the same care. Cardiac and pain management care are two areas that have been shown to have the largest gap in proper patient care.

According to the **National Institutes of Health (NIH)**, the origins of this issue stem back decades. Medical science used to be based on the thought that male and female physiology only varied because of sex and reproductive organs, which is not the case. For this reason, research was generally only conducted on males, as well as male tissue. This increased knowledge on how disease affects males, but left women neglected and misunderstood. This problem has been addressed. According to the NIH, women now make up 50% of participants in NIH research. This will continue to increase knowledge on how disease affects those differently based on their sex. Women's physiology is becoming better understood. Researchers are gaining knowledge on how gender affects physiology, metabolism, as well as symptoms and manifestation of disease. This will hopefully help physicians, as well as other healthcare providers provide better care to female patients.

Gender biases can have a whole host of consequences. Knowledge gaps are a huge one. As discussed below, a lack of research has led physicians to have a far better understanding of male physiology than women's. There is also a lack of women leadership in healthcare. A study done on the implicit gender bias among United States resident physicians found that a majority of people view men as naturally better leaders. Delayed diagnoses are a major consequence of gender bias and one that can severely impact patients. When doctors inevitably do not take a patient's symptoms seriously, it prevents them from receiving the correct diagnoses. In some cases it can take years to receive the correct diagnosis and treatment. A study conducted in Denmark in 2019 found that in "75% of cases, women waited longer on average for a diagnosis than men". Along the same lines, these biases can lead to inadequate symptom management which can prevent patients from receiving the proper medications to manage their symptoms. Specifically, women with chronic pain are often dismissed and not prescribed necessary medications to manage their pain. These issues can lead to women having a lack of trust in medical care. These biases can also lead to higher rates of women dying through illnesses such as heart attacks since there is a lack of awareness, and belief about how heart attacks affect women differently than men.

Accessing Healthcare as a Nonbinary or Transgender Individual

According to the CDC, it is estimated that 1.8 percent of high school students openly identify as transgender. This statistic does not include the amount of youth that identify as nonbinary. Of all adults in the United States, it is estimated that 0.6% identify as transgender or non binary. Meaning 1.4 million transgender and nonbinary people struggle to access essential resources. This is a major public health issue. It is estimated that 54% of transgender youth have attempted suicide, and 21% of reported some sort of self mutilation. 50% of transgender people have injected themselves with hormones that were obtained illegally. Making resources available to all transgender and nonbinary individuals is essential, for both their physical and mental health.

Once a person decides to seek care, they are hit by a wall of hurdles, including stigma and discrimination from the healthcare system. On top of this, legal, economic and social obstacles are often an issue. A recent qualitative study, conducted by *JAMA, the Journal of the American Medical Association*, looked at transgender and nonbinary youth and young adults, ages 9 to 24 years old and their experiences accessing healthcare. The findings of this study sadly showed that much needs to change. Healthcare for transgender youth is complex as most decisions have to be made before the age of independent medical consent. Puberty blockers, alongside hormone therapy are the most common gender affirming treatments. These are most beneficial when taken before the start of puberty. This becomes a challenge, as youth are underage and unable to begin the intervention without their parents' consent. If a parent refuses to consent, they are blocking their child from receiving treatment. Puberty cannot be reversed. Therefore a child will be impacted by their parent's decision for the rest of their life.

There is also a mix of contradicting information about healthcare procedures. The American Medical Association and the American Academy of Pediatrics endorse gender confirming treatments for teens, however medical guidelines still recommend against any gender reassignment surgery for individuals under the age of 18. This results in a limited number of surgeons performing pediatric gender reassignment surgeries. Before surgery, physicians generally use a set of mental health evaluations to ensure that their patients have an understanding of themselves and that medical intervention is the right answer. While most physicians believe that these evaluations are essential before beginning any gender affirming treatments, there has been criticism as some look at it as a "gate-keeping" measure and that it forces individuals to feel as though they have to prove that they are "trans enough".

For youth, parents' lack of approval and consent is one of the most common and life altering barriers, but sadly, even with parents on board, there are several other barriers that transgender individuals of all ages face. For one, many transgender individuals avoid seeking care in fear of humiliation, or being misunderstood. Once seeking care, insurance is a common barrier. Finding trans-friendly providers within a network can be a huge struggle. Even once a provider is found, waitlists tend to be several months to years long. Once receiving an appointment, many families struggle with getting their insurance to cover common treatment, such as hormone blockers.

It is evident that our healthcare system needs to change. Insurance is one of the most prominent barriers to care that transgender individuals face. However, in recent years, there has been a shift in the nation's legal position regarding coverage for members of the LGBTQ community. Under the Affordable Care Act's Section 1557, insurance companies are no longer able to raise rates based on one's gender identity. The decision by the Supreme Court in the Bostock vs. Clayton County case was another milestone for the transgender community. This decision made it a violation of the Title VII of the Civil Rights Act for an employer to fire individuals based off of their sexual orientation or gender identity. While there are still some gaps in coverage, especially when it comes to self-funded employers, these cases have begun to improve access to care for transgender individuals.

Changes within medical practices are also essential for improving patients' access, as well as comfort receiving medical care. Many relate to effective communication with patients. It is essential to refer to all patients using their preferred name and pronoun. Having questions on registration forms related to gender identity, such as fields for sex at birth, alongside preferred name and pronouns is an easy way to avoid misgendering patients. Alongside this, entering all given information into an electronic health record is a step that can be taken so that all staff are aware of a patient's preferred name and pronouns. If a physician is unaware of a patient's pronouns, the doctor should politely ask the patient how they would like to be addressed. If mistakes are made, apologies should immediately be made to the patient. If forms such as insurance forms, registration forms, and medical records have different names/sexes listed, and do not match, the doctor or administrator should discuss it with the patient in a straightforward, polite and private way. Doctors and front desk staff should not use the term "real" name. Some other tips are to only discuss a patient's transgender status in a private setting, not to ever joke about their gender identity, and to continue to use their preferred pronouns and name even when they are not present in the clinic.

In terms of adapting policies, procedures and facilities to be a more inclusive space, there are a variety of steps that clinics can take. For one, offering single occupancy bathrooms for all genders, as well as implementing policies to allow individuals to use the restroom that matches their gender identity is essential. Adding trans-friendly signage is a small step that can immediately make a difference in one's mindset within a facility. Actively hiring transgender people, and creating a channel for complaints and questions as well as implementing training for both new and old employees surrounding patient centered care for transgender individuals is also an essential step is improving our healthcare experience. Lastly, offering a full range of services to transgender patients, such as hormone therapy, HIV testing/prevention, support groups and employment opportunities, as well as having lists of other clinics and providers can help make transgender patients feel more comfortable seeking care.

Addressing biases in healthcare
Awareness is essential in addressing and helping to eliminate this specific bias in healthcare. Few physicians purposely deliver different care to patients based on gender. It is unconscious but can be changed with awareness, as well as education. The NIH offers courses specifically on sex and gender differences in medicine. These courses can be found at www.nih.org/women and are open to the public.

Finally, Denise Davis, a professor of medicine at the University of California, San Francisco offers these tips to help clinicians identify and fight gender biases

1. Diverse health care teams - Encourage staff to discuss gender bias and be comfortable having open discussions

2. Open ended questions - Encourage physicians to use open ended questions. Questions with limited possible responses are easier to be "contaminated by bias".

3. Substitution - If one feels as though they are being biased, they should be encouraged to think about what questions they would ask the patient if they were of a different gender. This will help limit assumptions and missed opportunities to gain essential information about patients.

4. Data collection and analysis - Data should be collected and analyzed in regards to gender differences to avoid issues that would otherwise go undetected

5. Checklists and guidelines - Standardized checklists, prompts and questions should be used for patients of all genders to ensure all patients are evaluated equally

6. Training opportunities - Offer training and bring in experts and coaches to talk to attending physicians and residents about patient communication to help clinicians become better aware of their own biases and ways to combat them.

Chapter Nine

The Impact of a Patient's Socioeconomic Status

By Dima Bischoff-Hashem, Julianna Celestin, and Airiana Michelle Davis

This chapter will focus on how the socioeconomic status of a patient impacts their perception of patient centered care. Utilizing the medical sociology approach and using the Social Determinants of Health as the basis. it further examines how the level of income of a patient can impact their role as a patient and their interaction with providers and facilities.

What is Socioeconomic Status?
According to the principles set by the American Psychological Association, socioeconomic status is defined as the social standing and [or] class of an individual or group. Socioeconomic status encompasses not only just income; but also, educational attainment, financial security, and subjective perceptions of social status and social class. It is utilized to describe the standing of an individual and [or] group of individuals compared to others. Socioeconomic status is divided into three levels known as low, middle, and high.

Socioeconomic Status and Access to Healthcare
Socioeconomics refers to society-related economic factors. These factors relate to and significantly influence one another. For instance, your employment will dictate your income. Your income level often correlates with your level of education and your level of education helps to dictate your employment. Thus, an endless cycle. A patient's socioeconomic status

significantly affects their ability to access healthcare and its resources. Research has shown that significant socioeconomic status health discrepancies exist. According to a study conducted on racial disparities in medical spending, healthcare expenditures for black and white households illustrated a bi-directional relationship between wealth and health. It emphasized that lower economic status leads to poorer health, which leads to a dangerous cycle of further impoverishment. For families of lower socioeconomic status, medical expenditures represent a significant financial burden that can make it challenging for families to acquire other goods and services.

A study conducted by Developmental Psychology indicated that socioeconomic status affects family stability, parenting practices, and developmental outcomes for children.

Socioeconomic status is a vital source of health inequity, as there is a significant correlation between socioeconomic status and health. In Chapter 2, we provided a brief explanation of how socioeconomic status and [or] economic security affects health.

Socioeconomic status in the United States is related to health outcomes. Individuals with a higher socioeconomic status typically have better health outcomes and resources relative to healthcare than those of lower socioeconomic status. Those living in lower income have health problems that are correlated to the lack of access to healthcare, food scarcity, poor nutrition, and environmental conditions in living and [or] workplaces.

The Impact of Health insurance on Health Care
While having limited access to healthcare, low socioeconomic status individuals describe a variety of ways in which they feel they had received an overall lower quality of care. A major factor is health insurance. A study conducted by the *Journal of Health Economics* compared private insurance holders of higher socioeconomic status to low socioeconomic status

patients. The study showed that low socioeconomic status patients are subjected to encountering different prescription and treatment options, and the reluctance of healthcare providers to administer treatment at all. Furthermore, lower socioeconomic status individuals often do not have adequate health care and are more prone to resorting to emergency departments for care, while their high socioeconomic counterparts have access to primary physicians and specialist care. Thus, this clearly illustrates that the type of healthcare insurance plan plays a significant role in receiving and accessing healthcare resources.

Furthermore, socioeconomic status affects health in terms of resources, which relates to limited access to care. An individual might have limited access to care as a result of being uninsured or underinsured and also be a distance from healthcare facilities. In addition, without financial security, an individual must decide what they can give up to seek medical care. They often need to decide whether going to seek care will mean lost wages, and if there is money available in the household to pay the insurance co-payments and for medication. And then there is the concern of receiving a bill from the doctor or healthcare facility when there is no insurance or the patient is underinsured.

Socioeconomic status also influences healthcare and the type of insurance individuals can afford. Low socioeconomic status is a crucial determinant of access to health care. Black, Indigenous, and People of Color (BIPOC) and low-income families are more prone to be uninsured and [or] on Medicaid, which is not widely accepted by many healthcare providers, especially private clinics and [or] specialists. Expensive healthcare services have disincentivized patients from visiting doctors with an emergency in fear of having to make out-of-pocket payments.

A Story About the Challenges of Access
In a written statement, mother Nicole Smith-Holt shared the story of her adult son with diabetes, who passed away because he could not afford insulin. Alec Raeshawn Smith, Nicole's son, was diagnosed with Type 1 diabetes in 2015 at the age of 24. Following the shocking news, he met with a dietitian and a diabetes specialist to make lifestyle changes that would protect his health and ensure that he could continue to be a healthy and present father for his young daughter. When Alec turned 26, he was no longer allowed to stay on his mother's health insurance and since his job didn't provide him with insurance nor could he afford his own, he had to pay the full, uninsured cost. Sadly, Alec only lived 27 days after losing his mother's health coverage. When he went to fill his prescription, it was $1,300, $300 more than he expected, and since he didn't have enough money, he left the pharmacy without it. A week later, he was found dead due to Diabetic Ketoacidosis. Nicole shares the story of her son's tragic passing as she advocates for affordable insulin, which would have saved his life.

Treatment Plans and Prescription Drug Costs
The medical dictionary defines a course of treatment or treatment plan as "a detailed plan with information about a patient's disease, the goal of treatment, the treatment options for the disease and possible side effects, and the expected length of treatment." Treatment plans often include prescribing medications, which patients have to take for a determined length of time. Prescription drugs are notoriously unaffordable in the United States because pharmaceutical prices go unregulated by the Food and Drug Administration (FDA), and therefore, those who are not financially stable often struggle to pay for essential medications.

Kaiser Health News states that one out of five Americans who are prescribed a drug cannot afford to fill their prescription. Name brand drugs are particularly expensive. In the United States, drug patents last for twenty years, meaning that after a drug company gets a patent on a medication, it can sell that drug for twenty years without competition from other companies. Since prescription medications are often necessary and life-saving, customers will pay almost any cost for them. Essentially, prescription medications have inelastic demand, so drug companies with patents can continue to raise prices on their products, a practice commonly known as price gouging. Low-income individuals are often uninsured meaning they are disproportionately harmed by high drug prices. While those with insurance only have to pay the copay for their prescriptions, uninsured individuals have to pay the full price. In fact, the Centers for Disease Control and Prevention found that 34 percent of uninsured adults in the country did not follow their doctor's dosage recommendation for financial reasons

Patients Prioritizing Choices
According to a PubMed article, healthcare practice includes situations in which choices and decisions are made, which offers opportunities for patients to exercise their options and for practitioners to respect those choices. So, respecting the patient's choice is a way to recognize their moral status as individuals and their capacity for self-determination. In Chapter 14, we will further explore the right of self-determination, which defines the right and ability to make your own decisions and choices about medical care and treatment received. However, unfortunately, respect for self-determination or autonomy is not an absolute principle within the healthcare system.

Maslow's Hierarchy of Needs is an approach to prioritizing patient needs. Maslow suggested that humans have basic everyday necessities such as physiological needs to survive, security needs for health and employment safety, social needs of family and friends, need for esteem, and a need for self-actualization. If given choices, patients would prioritize effective communication, location of care, trust in the provider, educational attainment, shared decision-making, quality of clinical care, access to health insurance, affordable treatment, and availability. Identifying what matters most to patients is essential for patient-centered care.

Studies have shown that distinctness in demographics and socioeconomic status leads to differences in a patient's health-related values and beliefs. Thus, the provider must understand their patient's demographics, allowing them to better provide adequate care and treatments to the patient. A study called *Patients' Priorities for Medical Care* studied the priorities for care among 225 patients. The respondents were given the following choices from which to choose their priorities as patients: continuity, coordination, comprehensiveness, availability, convenience, cost, expertise, and compassion. The results indicated that continuity of care was the highest priority among the participants. It was also discovered that patients with acute problems prioritize coordination and expertise, but patients with chronic illness prioritize continuity. Patients under 30 value coordination, while older patients value continuity and comprehensiveness. One example is a patient who lives up to three hours away from a health clinic of any kind, and their medical history indicates susceptibility to a chronic health disease. As a result, the patient's ability to receive effective immediate care is affected.

Therefore, it is important for healthcare providers to be culturally competent. When providers understand patient demographics, they can make better decisions based on patient needs. The future of our healthcare system is patient-centered care, which relies on having the correct information to understand challenges and refine our practices.

Chapter Ten

The Impact of Where a Patient Lives
By Aaliyah Anaya and Faalik Zahra

This chapter will explore if where a patient lives affects the level of care they receive. We examine experiences of patients living in suburban areas versus urban areas, as well as the experiences of those who are indigent. The chapter focuses on the level of access based on the neighborhood of the patient and how other factors such as income level, education, and social support affect a patient's access to care and the level of patient centered care.

The Patient Experience in Urban Areas
Urban areas are home to approximately 62.7% of the American population, according to the United States Census Bureau. There are a variety of reasons for the influx to urban areas. Cities often have higher-paying jobs, public transportation, entertainment, higher education, and typically the major healthcare facilities and teaching hospitals. Healthcare organizations in urban environments have several advantages over those based in rural areas due to greater access to state-of-the art medical equipment and the top providers in the area. Because urban areas have a more diverse population, they also have a higher representation of healthier and more affluent residents. This population has a high percentage of private sector insurance coverage, which pays higher rates than public programs such as Medicare and Medicaid. People with basic economic and lifestyle advantages

living in an urban area are desirable to many healthcare professionals. From a patient perspective, access to health care services tends to be better in urban areas, which increases the likelihood of completing annual wellness visits, receiving regular care, and monitoring chronic conditions. This, in turn, leads to better health outcomes and lower total cost of care.

Urban areas are home to approximately 62.7% of the American population, according to the United States Census Bureau. There are a variety of reasons for the influx to urban areas. Cities often have higher-paying jobs, public transportation, entertainment, higher education, and healthcare. Healthcare organizations in urban environments have several advantages over those based in rural areas due to greater access to state-of-the art medical equipment and the top providers in the area.. Because urban areas have a more diverse population, they also have a higher representation of healthier and more affluent residents. This population has a high percentage of private sector insurance coverage, which pays higher rates than public programs such as Medicare and Medicaid. People with basic economic and lifestyle advantages of an urban area are desirable to many healthcare professionals. From a patient perspective, access to health care services tends to be better in urban areas, which increases the likelihood of completing annual wellness visits, receiving regular care, and monitoring chronic conditions. This, in turn, leads to better health outcomes and lower total cost of care.

The migration to urban areas means more people are accounted for when healthcare delivery systems complete community needs assessments. This enables more social determinants to be addressed for more people.

The Patient Experience for the Homeless

Conversely, people experiencing homelessness are frequently marginalized and face barriers to receiving accessible healthcare services. Simply being without a home is associated with enormous health inequalities, with homelessness being a key driver of poor health. It is therefore critical to treat homelessness as a combined health and social issue in order to improve the health outcomes of the homeless. The National Health Care for the Homeless Council reports that homeless people are three to six times more likely to become ill than those who live in some type of dwelling. Unfortunately, many homeless people who are ill and need treatment never receive medical care. Barriers to healthcare include lack of knowledge of where to get treated, lack of access to transportation, and lack of identification. The most common obstacle is the cost. As a result, many homeless people utilize hospital emergency rooms as their primary source of healthcare. Not only is this not the most effective form of care for homeless people since it provides little continuity, but it is also very expensive for hospitals and the government.

There is significant evidence that shows a strong association between homelessness and health disadvantage. In the homeless population, the Social Determinants of Health often start with adverse early life experiences followed by poor educational outcomes and disengagement, involvement with drugs, unstable work history, and often imprisonment. It is these circumstances and a lack of a stable support network that leads to homelessness.

Several programs have been developed to provide health care services to homeless people. Federally funded programs, such as the Health Care for the Homeless Council, are designed to provide primary health care to homeless persons. These programs are required to provide primary health care, substance abuse services, emergency care, outreach, and assistance in qualifying for housing. The lack of affordable housing complicates efforts to provide healthcare to homeless persons. Housing is the first form of treatment for homeless people with medical problems, protecting them against illness and making it possible for those who are ill to recover. Shelter-based clinics provide the types of services most frequently found throughout the country, serving the homeless population. Rescue missions serve the homeless for extended periods of time and have substantial access to networks with healthcare services, housing, and social services. These clinics tend to be staffed by volunteer doctors and nurses that rely heavily on private donations. However, because of the religious aspects of the organizations that operate these clinics, many homeless people are not willing to go to them.

Housing has long been recognized as a basic human right and a core social determinant of health. Universal access to affordable, high-quality, and comprehensive health care is essential in the fight to end homelessness. The goal should be to enable homeless people to have access to the range of services that already exist, thereby decreasing their need for specialized services.

Healthcare Facilities in Low-Income Neighborhoods
Patients who live in poor areas are more likely to have health problems and experience limited access to healthcare. Hospital closures have increased throughout the country, and the communities with the greatest shortage of health facilities tend to be the areas with the highest poverty. These facilities in poor areas tend to treat most patients on Medicare, Medicaid, or with no insurance, which is a challenge related to reimbursement and patient communication. Even with insurance, these patients tend to face longer wait times and delays in care. It is evident that hospital and practice closures in poor areas reduce access to care.

Patients who live in cities are not always guaranteed better access to health care, particularly those who live in low-income neighborhoods. They are less likely to have jobs, transportation, and access to healthy food. Many providers and hospitals leave poor areas, which have the greatest healthcare needs, to follow privately insured patients in wealthier areas. As the presence of healthcare facilities in low-income neighborhoods decreases, a growing number of evidence shows that poor people are more likely to be in poor health. It is higher-income areas, where people are healthier and mobile that are most likely to get new health facilities. The supply of healthcare providers in poor neighborhoods is often affected by the lack of medical laboratories or medical supply companies which all act as barriers and drive up the cost of operating a facility.

To some extent, income and wealth directly support better overall health because wealthier people can afford the resources and services within their neighborhoods. Wealthy environments have more access to green space, recreational programs, and facilities for regular exercising and active living.

The Bottom Line – The Effect of Where the Patient Lives on Healthcare Access

Where a patient lives plays a crucial role in an individual's life. Depending on the area where the individual resides can greatly affect the person they become and the beliefs that they develop.

Patients are often unaware of their circumstance as compared to other areas. This can make it hard to identify this as an issue that must be handled by the patient. Providers should also be aware of the area that the facility is located at to ensure that they are able to better cater to the demographic. The goal of all facilities and all providers should be to only enhance the quality of care that the patient receives and not hinder their experience.

The placement of facilities leads has a direct effect on the experiences of patients. If an area has more facilities, then there are more professionals to access and less stress on the professionals to provide care. Providers can then spend more time with patients and are less stressed while doing so, improving the treatment that the patients receive. When the facilities are fewer in number and harder to access by transportation, it becomes difficult for many patients to get the care they need and are entitled to.

Patients that reside in urban areas have more access to healthcare professionals. Often these are areas with more people leading to more healthcare facilities existing there. More healthcare facilities increase the option of care that the patient receives while also indirectly increasing the quality of the care that the facility may provide. The more facilities that are present in a given area will increase competition among the various facilities thereby causing them to better the services they provide. It will also increase the patient's accessibility to healthcare facilities. The increased exposure causes the patient to feel more confident and educated when visiting a healthcare facility. Patients in rural areas may have a similar experience with healthcare professionals and facilities.

However, rural areas have fewer facilities, and it may take longer to travel to them, which often can create problems in an emergency. However, studies have shown that those living in rural areas compensate for the fewer amount of facilities by living close to the facilities that do exist. Finally, as we have mentioned, one of the most challenging problems in terms of providing patient centered care to a population, based on where a patient lives, is the case of the homeless individual

It is therefore clear that where a patient lives can very much affect their access to healthcare services and the quality of care they receive, and their experiences as a patient. Healthcare facilities are paying attending to population trends, and trying to meet the needs of all patients, by placing smaller hospitals and medical offices closer to where these facilities are most needed. That is one of the reasons that in recent years, there has been an increase in urgent care and emergent care facilities being built, especially in urban areas and low-income neighborhoods.

Chapter Eleven

The Impact of a Patient's Social Circle
By Faalik Zahra

This chapter will focus on how the social circle of a patient impacts their perception of patient-centered care. Social circles are a significant aspect of an individual's life and perception of their world. Different social experiences lead to different healthcare expectations. These expectations lead to varying ideals regarding how patient-centered care should be performed. The chapter will delve deeper into these beliefs to showcase how different social circles can lead to particular perceptions of patient-centered care.

Definitions

Social Circle: Individuals who one interacts with frequently.

Perceptions: Using previous experiences and beliefs as a way to understand future events and instances

Where Patients Gain Their Knowledge of Healthcare

Knowledge is received through a variety of different sources, whether from friends, the internet, or daily interactions with co-workers, family, and others. According to a study performed by Carolyn Cutili, most patients believe that the most trusted source of healthcare information is their healthcare providers. Interactions between healthcare professionals and patients often occur within healthcare facilities including medical offices. But some of the social interactions with a provider occur outside of the conventional healthcare facility. The growing technological advancements of medicine have allowed patients to utilize telemedicine to interact with providers from their homes. Others may contact healthcare professionals that they know personally through their social circle. And so, patients who have healthcare workers in their social circle have increased access to knowledge regarding healthcare and various medical procedures.

Having a Healthcare Professional in Your Social Circle

According to the CDC, there are over 18 million healthcare workers in the United States. These healthcare workers are influencing the patient population not only in healthcare facilities, but personally as well. People often will utilize their personal relationships to understand more about their medical circumstances and relieve any stress they may have regarding their health. Patients will often discuss their medical condition with their contact before they visit their primary physician or other healthcare professional. It assists in easing their stress and allows them to feel prepared for their visit. By talking to a social contact who is in healthcare, allows the patient to understand what questions to ask and be better prepared to be receptive to what is said to them. Having healthcare professionals in your social circle allows individuals to become more educated on various topics involving the individual's health. Having a trusted friend who is a doctor, a nurse, a rehab therapist, a mental health professional, or a physician assistant is valuable in preparing a patient for a visit to their healthcare provider. However, it is common for the good friend, who happens to be in healthcare, to caution the patient and remind them that the person they need to get the final answer from is their healthcare provider. As patients, we should not be offended by this response, since we need to appreciate that legally our chosen healthcare providers need to be the ones we discuss our treatment approach with, and that our friends in healthcare are there to simply answer some initial questions, and not to diagnose.

Not Having a Healthcare Professional in Your Social Circle

Patients without personal connections in the healthcare industry interact with healthcare professionals solely during their visits to the clinic or other facility. These patients rely heavily on their primary physician for any medical attention they may need. In most circumstances, this interaction is sufficient for patients to feel treated and educated. For patients, this may be the only healthcare professional that they communicate with, thus encouraging them to disclose all their concerns to them.

Patients may often feel stressed because they want to make sure that they receive all the information necessary during their visit. If this is the first time they hear about a particular illness or circumstance, it can also become challenging to know what questions to ask. When something is not fully understood during their visit, the patient must contact their provider again to understand it. Therefore, many patients turn to friends and family who perhaps have had similar healthcare experiences to learn what they might expect before seeing their doctor. At the same time, many patients turn to the internet and begin to research what they think could be wrong with them, and this often is very dangerous and can cause great anxiety and needless worry. Consulting "Dr. Google" is often generally not a good idea.

Who We Socialize With Can Impact Our Perceptions of Healthcare Delivery

Often, patients with interactions with social contacts in the healthcare field will feel increasingly confident and educated while visiting the healthcare facility. They may have already obtained a second opinion on the diagnosis or have heard of the procedure from their friend who is a doctor or a nurse or a physician assistant. Patients without healthcare professionals in their social circle may be hesitant to do so because they usually will not trust someone more than their primary physician. These patients place a higher emphasis on their visits to the healthcare facilities and usually ensure they receive all necessary information during their time there. For those without healthcare providers in their social network, the comfort of knowing that they can call a friend later to further elaborate on their circumstance is not an option. Indirectly this can impact their relationship with healthcare because now, the only time they interact with professionals is for a routine check-up or due to an emergency situation. Physical and mental health can be highly personal, motivating individuals to ask healthcare professionals within their social circle first. They have that comfort with that individual, which makes the task seem less daunting. Then when visiting a physician at the clinic, they are more comfortable because they are already aware of the issue and have some knowledge of the topic—ultimately leading them to ask more questions making the session more productive and beneficial for the individual.

Overall, whether a patient has healthcare professionals within their social circle or not, typically will not impact the care that they are receiving. It may lead to different experiences because of the knowledge that the individual has. Our social network influences our thoughts, our beliefs, our preferences, and our education and understanding about healthcare.

When a friend or family member shares a story about their patient experience with us, it can impact how we perceive the quality of care that one receives at a given hospital or healthcare provider, and those influences become extremely important in our overall perception of which providers we choose and what facilities we wish to use when we need to be hospitalized or need to access an urgent care center, or we need blood work done or imaging done. Our social circle definitely influences our perception of what constitutes good patient centered care, as well as our reasonable expectations of the healthcare system.

Chapter Twelve

The Impact of a Patient's Access to Healthcare
By Courtney Pokallus

Often when thinking about quality healthcare, you immediately think about how you personally are treated as a patient. Our perception of quality healthcare focuses on how doctors, nurses and other staff treat us, and if they are kind and compassionate. It also includes how well the treatment they suggest works to resolve our health concerns. Most of us do not equate quality healthcare with our access to healthcare, but access is just as important, if not more important.

Access to Care
So why is the issue of access to healthcare so important, and why is it so essential to patient centered care? The Office of Disease Prevention and Health Promotion (ODPHP) outlines two indicators that defines whether a person has good access to healthcare. The first is if the person has medical insurance and the second is if the person has a primary care physician.

If you don't have healthcare insurance, accessing healthcare services can be extremely expensive and usually diverts individuals from seeking care. In 2020, 8.6% of the population of the United States or about 28 million people did not have any form of health insurance. Without proper medical insurance, a patient's access to specialists, tests, surgeries, and in some cases, the hospitals they can choose becomes limited and very challenging. In some cases, lack of insurance can lead to worsening conditions and in some cases, even death because the proper diagnosis has not been made and/or the treatment for the illness could not be implemented properly.

Having a primary care physician is also very important for overall health. Having a PCP ensures that a patient has yearly checkups where, even if the patient is completely healthy, the patient is connecting with a healthcare provider to help with any health concerns and identify any health risks.

The Important Role of the Primary Care Provider (PCP)

The OCPHP points out that primary care providers (PCPs) play an important role in protecting the health and safety of the communities they serve. PCPs develop meaningful and sustained relationships with patients and provide integrated services while practicing in the context of family and community. Having a usual PCP ensures a greater patient trust in the provider, better communication between provider and patient, and an increased likelihood that patients will receive appropriate care. In addition, having access to healthcare can prevent disease and disability, detect and treat illnesses or other health conditions, increase quality of life, reduce the likelihood of premature (early) death and increase life expectancy.

The Five Dimensions of Access

Another way to define access to healthcare is with the *International Journal for Equity and Health's* Five Dimensions of Access.

These five dimensions include
1) approachability
2) acceptability
3) availability and accommodation
4) affordability
5) appropriateness

These points are very important not only to ensure quality access to healthcare, but also for the overall comfort of the patient. Thinking about yourself going to a doctor with concerns about your health, would you want to be seen by a physician that did not provide you with these five points? We want our healthcare providers to be approachable, accepting of who we are and how we live our lives, available when we need them, affordable, and appropriate in their conversations with us and in the decisions they make regarding our care.

How Do the Social Determinants of Health Affect Access to Care?

As explained in Chapter 2, the Social Determinants of Health are the external conditions that very much influence a person's health status. The World Health Organization does an excellent job of describing the social determinants of health and explaining why they are important.

"The Social Determinants of Health (SDH) are the non-medical factors that influence health outcomes. They are the conditions in which people are born, grow, work, live, and age, and the wider set of forces and systems shaping the conditions of daily life. These forces and systems include economic policies and systems, development agendas, social norms, social policies and political systems. The SDH have an important influence on health inequities - the unfair and avoidable differences in health status seen within and between countries. In countries at all levels of income, health and illness follow a social gradient: the lower the socioeconomic position, the worse the health."

The following is a list of the Social Determinants of Health that influence health equity in positive and negative ways:

- Income and social protection
- Education
- Unemployment and job insecurity
- Working life conditions
- Food insecurity

- Housing, basic amenities and the environment
- Early childhood development
- Social inclusion and non-discrimination
- Structural conflict
- Access to affordable health services of decent quality

Research shows that the social determinants can be more important in influencing our overall health than the care a patient receives or lifestyle choices we make. For example, numerous studies suggest that SDH accounts for between 30-55% of health outcomes. In addition, estimates show that the contribution of sectors outside health to population health outcomes exceeds the contribution from the health sector.

WHO points out that "addressing the SDH appropriately is fundamental for improving health and reducing longstanding inequities in health, which requires action by all sectors and civil society. The Social Determinants of Health are crucial to a patient's access to healthcare. Where the person lives, their income level, their education etc. has a huge impact on the access to healthcare they will receive, as has been explored in other chapters in this book.

Defining Patient Centered Care
Now that I have touched on what access to healthcare is, it is time to talk about patient-centered care. Patient centered care can be defined in many different ways. My favorite definition and the one I think is most true is **patients actively participating in their own medical treatment**. This is very important to many patients and families of patients to ensure that they are getting what they want out of their care and that it works best for their needs. The individuality of patient-centered care is something that creates a strong patient-provider relationship as each patient is treated as an individual. Each patient's treatment is catered specifically for each patient.

The World Health Organization also has created an excellent informative definition for patient-centered care.

"The overall vision for people-centered health care is one in which individuals, families and communities are served by and are able to participate in trusted health systems that respond to their needs in humane and holistic ways. The health system is designed around stakeholder needs and enables individuals, families and communities to collaborate with health practitioners and health care organizations in the public, private and not-for-profit health and related sectors in driving improvements in the quality and responsiveness of health care.

People-centered health care is rooted in universally held values and principles which are enshrined in international law, such as human rights and dignity, nondiscrimination, participation and empowerment, access and equity, and a partnership of equals. It aims to achieve better outcomes for individuals, families, communities, health practitioners, health care organizations and health systems by promoting the following:

- ***Culture of care and communication***. Health care consumers being informed and involved in decision-making and having choices; providers showing respect for their privacy and dignity and responding to their needs in a holistic manner.

- ***Responsible, responsive and accountable services and institutions***. Providing affordable, accessible, safe, ethical, effective, evidence-based and holistic health care.

- ***Supportive health care environments***. Putting in place appropriate policies and interventions, positive care and work environments, strong primary care workforce, and mechanisms for stakeholders' involvement in health services planning, policy development and feedback for quality improvement"(WHO).

Patient-centered care is so important to making the patient feel safe and comfortable in any type of healthcare office. Going to a hospital or physician's office is scary and uncomfortable for many people. Maintaining a patient-centered practice helps these patients feel more in control of their care.

How Does Access to Care Impact Patient Centered Care?

So, here is the bottom line. How does patient-centered care influence a patient's access to healthcare? It is first important to understand that just because a person has access to healthcare - a primary care physician and health insurance – it does not mean that they receive quality healthcare. There are so many stories of people who have had medical issues that are not treated correctly or with compassion. This makes the situation harder and more stressful for the patient who just wants to be treated for their health concerns. So many people go from specialist to specialist to find out what is causing their pain and discomfort and are not given answers by any of the doctors they visit. Instead they get what has become known as the "specialist runaround". This is frustrating and very demoralizing for any patient. There are so many examples of how having basic access to healthcare does not correlate to having *quality* access to healthcare. And that is where patient-centered care comes in. As stated before, patient-centered care is giving the patient a role to play in their own treatment. This means letting a patient have a say in how they want to be treated. It also means being a compassionate physician to the patient and really hearing their concerns and listening to how they feel. Listening to the patient describe symptoms and emotions is what gives physicians the best information they need to treat a patient.

Let's look at two studies that examine the connection between access to care and patient centered care. Both of these studies are available through the National Library of Medicine. The first study is called *The Impact of Patient-Centered Care on Outcomes* by M. Stewart, J. Brown, A. Donner, I. R. McWhinney, J. Oates, W. W. Weston, and J. Jordan. This study is affiliated with the Centre for Studies in Family Medicine, The University of Western Ontario, London, Canada. In this study, the researchers observed 39 physicians and 315 patients and looked for patient-centered communication. The patients were then asked questions about their visits. Their conclusions were reported in the following way:

"Patient-centered communication influences patients' health through perceptions that their visit was patient centered, and especially through perceptions that common ground was achieved with the physician. Patient-centered practice improved health status and increased the efficiency of care by reducing diagnostic tests and referrals".

Looking at the results of this study, you can see that the patients felt more comfortable and better heard about their concerns when the physician used a patient-centered approach.

The second study is titled *Patient-Centered Care Factors and Access to Care: a Path Analysis Using the Andersen Behavior Model* by J.R. Hong, S.K. Samuels, J. H. Huo, N. Lee, H. Mansoor, and R. P. Duncan, affiliated with Department of Health Services Research, Management and Policy, College of Public Health and Health Professions, University of Florida, Gainesville, Florida. This study included 15.787 individuals with health insurance. They used a measurement tool called the Anderson Behavioral Model to determine the associations among usual source of care, travel time to provider, financial disadvantage, patient-centered care factors that are perceived with the health provider, shared decision-making, and value of health care), and access to care (perceived access to care and unmet need of health services). Their conclusions are as follows.

"Our findings suggest that better patient-centered care factors are associated with enhanced patient access to care. Efforts that focus on improving patient experience could be an effective approach along with coverage expansion to enhance access to quality care".

Looking at the results of this study, you can see that using a patient-centered approach gives patients a better quality experience and is associated with having better access to healthcare.

Using a patient-centered approach is important for so many reasons. The patients can tell when they are being treated with a patient-centered approach and when they are not. This approach gives them a feeling of comfort and compassion from the physician and overall helps give patients a better access to quality healthcare. Without patient-centered approaches being used by physicians and other healthcare providers, it can make the patient feel uncomfortable, and very often cause the patient to consider going to the doctor as a last resort instead of an important part of their overall healthcare treatment. Treating patients with compassion, really listening to their concerns, and individualizing the treatment they prefer will ultimately create a better outlook on the healthcare experience for the patient ultimately giving them a better access to healthcare with the knowledge that when they are stepping into a healthcare office they are respected and that their concerns will be treated with the highest standards.

Chapter Thirteen

The Impact of the Right to Self-Determination

By Dima Bischoff-Hashem and Airiana Michelle Davis

This chapter will explore the impact of the right of self-determination and how this right affects patient-centered care. Issues include reproductive rights, food consumption, use of medications, compliance with treatment plans, and the issue of vaccinations.

Self-Determination in Healthcare
Everyone wants the freedom to choose. A choice means individual autonomy or freedom, a concept that emerged in ethical theories. As patients, we have a legal right to make our own healthcare decisions. The right of self-determination implies the right and ability to make your own choices and decisions about medical care and treatment, as long as it's within legal boundaries. This law requires patients to be fit and competent for rational decision-making. Through legal documents such as the Living Will and the Durable Healthcare Power of Attorney, patients can also pre-determine the type of care the wish to receive even when they reach a situation that makes them incompetent, and no longer able to make their own medical decisions. The right of self-determination was given to us, as patients, in 1991 when Congress enacted the **Patient Self-Determination Act**. While focused on the right to use a Living Will or Durable Healthcare Power of Attorney when a patient can no longer verbalize their medical decisions, the act has been broadened to give patients the right to say no to a recommended treatment plan from their healthcare providers.

Self-Determination Theory states that people have three psychological needs for well-being and performance: relatedness, competence, and autonomy. We all have the need to feel affection or care, to feel effective in environments, and to feel that we are acting with a sense of control. Research indicates the importance of creating a supportive environment that satisfies all three needs. In addition, studies have shown that when providers give patients choices, it enhances patient self-determination and better informs them about their health conditions and treatments. Thus, the self-determination theory is relevant to implementing patient-centered care because health outcomes are optimized when practitioners and providers support patient autonomy, competence, and relatedness.

The Patient Self-Determination Act requires compliance, meaning providers must communicate with patients about healthcare options and protect their rights to self-determination. For example, a patient has the right to refuse to accept treatment or care based on morals, religious beliefs, or any other logical reason, and providers must support that patient. So, it is essential for providers not to be controlling their patients, meaning they should respect the medical decisions of their patients. Certainly, if a patient refuses treatment such as not agreeing to have recommended surgery or taking a certain prescribed medication, once the provider presents the patient with information on the risks of not complying, the patient has the right to refuse treatment. According to the *Journal for Nurse Practitioners*, healthcare providers can assist patients with options in rehabilitation treatments, rationales, voicing their own opinions, providing information for decision-making, providing feedback about progress, and encouraging family members to be supportive.

The Impact of Self-Determination on Reproductive Rights

Reproductive rights are human rights associated with sexual health, reproductive health, and autonomy. It recognizes that women are autonomous agents with authority to make sexual and reproductive decisions free from interference, discrimination, coercion, and violence. Reproductive rights are essential to women's socioeconomic well-being and overall health by protecting their dignity. Studies have shown that women who make their own decisions about their reproductive health have more excellent stability and satisfaction, which creates a better society and protects the environment from overpopulation. Without the right to reproductive self-determination, woman risk the lack of autonomy, unplanned pregnancies, the spread of HIV/AIDS, increased poverty, and undergoing unsafe medical procedures. So, providers must have an effective relationship with their patients to ensure safe treatments and healthy reproductive experiences in healthcare facilities. For example, a pregnant woman will go to the hospital because of mild contractions and dilations. When the provider examines the woman, they believe nothing is alarming; the baby isn't coming, and sends the woman back home. However, the woman stands firm about her pain levels and speaks up about her rights. So, the physician must trust and respect the woman's reasoning to help safely deliver the baby. Thus, a woman's effective exercise of her rights to reproductive self-determination depends entirely on equality in civil, cultural, economic, political, and social life. Therefore, the government must take the necessary measures to eradicate social and cultural patterns that perpetuate notions of women's inferiority. They should abolish traditional practices that harm children's health, including forced marriages, and ensure access to health services consistent with the child's evolving capacities.

The Impact of Self-Determination on Food Consumption

Food is a necessity for every living thing. Food is medicine because it can maintain, prevent, and treat diseases. Food consumption is a periodic behavior triggered at different moments of the day by various contributing factors like time, social context, and sensory stimulation. Self-determination in food consumption allows a patient to eat what they want, even it is against the suggestions of their healthcare provider. The food we eat gives our bodies the instructions and materials to function correctly. It is essential because healthy food consumption can help strengthen the immune system, improve blood circulation, reduce cardiovascular diseases, and prevent chronic illnesses. What we consume can have a significant impact on our health. So, choosing the proper diet for health is essential. Some easy ways for patients to make better health decisions include reviewing dietary guidelines, cooking smarter, purchasing low-fat and low-calorie foods, eating smaller portions, and being cautious when eating out. A unique approach to adopting a healthier habit is to eat intentionally, trying to research healthy meal plans, and buying the necessary food items at the grocery store. Access to safe and affordable foods that induce healthy food consumption supports the longevity of a patient. However, lack of accessibility to markets, poor availability of the healthiest foods, and lack of transportation to find healthy are constant barriers, which result in adverse health outcomes. So, while a patient may have the ability to find healthy food, if they choose not to eat that way, that is their decision.

Use of Medications

Self-determination can affect the patient's use of medication. Providers prescribe medicine to diagnose, treat, cure, or prevent diseases. The effectiveness of drugs is within the patient's control. Patients have the right to ask and understand the type of medications prescribed to them. The United States Food and Drug Administration (FDA) suggests that patients or family members ask questions about the name, the results, the effectiveness, symptoms, side effects, and safety of medications. Some factors contributing to patients refusing to use the medication are poor patient-provider relationships, lack of trust, communication, and understanding, cost, physical impairments, psychological barriers, and cultural biases. Since patients have the right to make their own decisions about using the medication, it could result in patients self-medicating. According to the World Health Organization (WHO), self-medication is the selected use of medicines to treat self-diagnosed disorders or illnesses or the continued use of drugs prescribed for chronic diseases. However, patients can risk misdiagnosing themselves, taking excessive medicine, and extend the time they take the medicine beyond when it is healthy to do so. Thus, patients must be honest about their medical history and speak up about their concerns during doctor visits. Therefore, providers must work with their patients to overcome these barriers, educate them, and monitor medication use to improve health outcomes.

Self-Determination and Compliance with Treatment Plans
In healthcare, a treatment plan is a guide or outline of therapeutic strategies that incorporate education, dietary adjustment, drug therapy, exercise program, and participation of health professionals for a patient. Compliance refers to the patient's adherence to the treatment plan and completion of care procedures and visits. A patient's compliance with their recommended treatment plan is essential because treatment plans help manage chronic illnesses. Often, treatment plans require a long duration of medication use. So, patient education and participation are necessary to set the right goals for treatment. The patient's capacity for understanding plays a factor in determining if they are competent and can make their own decisions.

When patients refuse medication or treatments, it needs to be determined if their concerns are logical and factual. Studies have shown that most patients will refuse to comply with treatments based on denial, fear, costs, misinformation, moral beliefs, ethical concerns, and physical and psychological burdens of treatment. Age is also sometimes a factor of a patient's unwillingness to comply with treatment plans, which can be associated with cognitive impairment or just plain stubbornness. Patients older than 65 living alone have lower compliance with taking medicine, changing their lifestyle, and keeping up with appointments. Despite age, patients still have the right to weigh their concerns about the risk of treatments and decide what is best for them. To improve patient compliance in healthcare, providers should implement treatment plans as a collaborative approach. Thus, providers should use the principle of informed consent when discussing the use of medications and treatment plans. Health professionals must also consider the patient's demographics, correct diagnosis, financial status, treatment goals, measurable objectives, interventions, timelines, frequency, and progress tracking. Multiple options for treatment plans allow patients to choose a primary and backup plan. However, some patients may not have the time, resources, or finances to try every treatment option. Therefore, alternative treatments like healing arts, acupuncture, chiropractic adjustments, and herbal medicines can often benefit a patient. These methods not only use medication to treat physical symptoms, but they also aim to treat the entire body along with the mind. Alternative treatment methods are often effective for a speedy recovery and improving patient care.

The Issue of Vaccinations
According to the World Health Organization, vaccinations are a simple, safe, and effective way of protecting people from harmful diseases before they come into contact with them. Vaccinations create antibodies and build resistance to specific infections in the body while strengthening our immune system. Vaccine hesitancy is about patients making their own choices. Online health information can empower patients to

participate in healthcare decisions, but cause many misconceptions and misunderstandings for a patient, especially with vaccinations. Individuals must choose between anti-vaccination or pro-vaccinations. False information about vaccines and their effects has caused patients to refuse vaccine treatment. Each vaccine has a different impact on everyone. Vaccinations can cause significant risks to specific individuals. For example, patients should not get the flu shot if they are severely ill, younger than six months old, pregnant, or have chronic diseases, a compromised immune system, egg allergies, or a prior life-threatening reaction.

For most people, vaccines are safe, but if a patient has concerns, they should talk to their doctor or provider for a different opinion. Thus, healthcare providers educating their patients about vaccines is vital. By sharing valuable information, providers can help build stronger relationships with their patients through trust and communication. According to the Centers for Disease Control (CDC), studies show that a solid recommendation from providers is significant in whether a patient decides to vaccinate. Other studies have indicated that reassuring communication does not increase vaccine acceptance or trust, leading to conspiracies because many want transparency and consistent information about vaccines. Today, many patients want transparency. Transparency can prevent uncertainty, even if it cannot eliminate the constant misinformation of science or increase vaccination acceptance. Many people must undergo vaccinations for a vaccine to help bring pandemics and epidemics under control. So, in these unprecedented times of the COVID-19 pandemic and the Monkeypox outbreak, patients need remarkable transparency.

The Social Determinants of Health and the Right to Self-Determination

All of the above areas of self-determination: reproductive rights, use of medication, issue of vaccinations, compliance with treatment plans, and food consumption, are impacted by social determinants of health. People's education, economic status, and other factors greatly influence their health decisions. For example, patients may make different decisions on vaccinations, medications, and food consumption if providers educate patients more on the effects of these things on their bodies. In addition, some people have no choice but to disregard their doctors' food and medication recommendations due to financial limitations.

Thus, every healthcare provider should comply to protect their patient's right to self-determination in every possible situation. Unfortunately, every patient does not receive the same health outcomes due to the impact of the Social Determinants of Health. The education of the patient, their income status, their marital status, their built environment, their community and social circle, and their economic stability all contribute to patient's decision-making. So, providers need to create an emotionally supportive environment that satisfies their patients' psychological needs to ensure their self-determination. Providers can help their patients by eliminating socio-economic barriers, advocating for patient rights, educating patients on health information, providing access to quality care, being transparent and timely about information, aligning their values with the patient's goals,
including the family's support, collaborating on decisions, prioritizing the patient's well-being, and overall respecting the patient's views, values, and choices. Accordingly, increased patient self-determination and health decision-making can result in a solid patient-provider relationship, improving patient-centered care. Health outcomes are optimized when providers support patient autonomy, competence, and relatedness.

PART FOUR
LIFE CYCLES

Chapter Fourteen

Birth to Adolescence
By Bob Kieserman and Courtney Pokallus

The birth of a baby is one of the most beautiful and happiest times of life for new parents. It can also be a frightening time, especially for first time parents, as they slowly gain confidence that they can care for this new little human being. When we look at the reasonable expectations of parents of a new baby from the perspective of caring for the medical needs of the child, there are many unique aspects to consider.

The first is probably that as a patient, the baby obviously has no expectations and it is the expectations of the parents that need to be met by the healthcare delivery system. The second is that legally a parent or legal guardian is responsible for making the decisions for their child until they reach the age of 18 years old. In the previous chapter, we learned about the right of self-determination. What we will discover as we explore the expectations of parents and patients from birth to adolescence is that the clear cut rule of who makes the medical decisions has some exceptions.

Birth to 12 Years Old
When a baby is born, every parent hopes that the delivery goes well and that there are no complications. Occasionally, a baby is born and needs some immediate intervention. A very specialized branch of pediatric medicine was created around 1960. It is called *neonatology*, and for those parents who have needed their babies to have the intervention of this specialist, they will agree that these doctors are true lifesavers. When a child is born premature or with a problem that needs to be addressed at birth, the neonatologist is there at the delivery table to go to work as soon as the baby is delivered. Through

many marvelous miracles of medical science, thousands of babies a year receive very special care in their first hours, days, and weeks of life, going on to have perfectly normal lives medically. So, in this situation, the major reasonable expectation of the mother giving birth and her partner is to be taken care of during the birthing process so that the birth has no complications and then taking care of the baby once the child has been delivered.

Medical Miracles
Before we move on, this is an ideal point to talk about an issue that has not yet been addressed in the book. It is quite relevant to what often happens in the hospital in the case of a premature or health compromised baby or really any patient that is in critical condition. As part of our exploration of patient centered care, we need to recognize the existence of medical miracles, and how they happen every day.

The prognosis of a patient may look very grim. The patient may be being kept alive with machines and in a natural coma, or medically-induced coma to keep the critical patient comfortable. The doctors and medical team have done everything they can to improve the patient's condition, but it is not looking good. All of a sudden, the patient begins to respond to the treatment, and the doctors are baffled. They cannot explain what has happened medically. This unexpected positive turn of events is attributed to what doctors call a medical miracle. Many studies have been conducted and many papers have been written about medical miracles, and they focus on one particular element that is very much a part of a patient's care, and that is prayer and religion. Whether the patient and the family are religious or not, it is a well documented fact that when all looks dismal, the family and friends of the patient typically turn to prayer, based on their own beliefs and their own connection with a Higher Power. Religious leaders often explain that when there is a crisis in a person's life, and even more so, a medical crisis, it is natural for most of us to reach out to our Higher Power to ask for help for ourselves if we are the patient or someone we care about. Medical sociologists very much believe this helps a patient, the family, and friends to cope better with the patient's critical state, but it is also believed and accepted by the medical profession that prayer and faith at this difficult time does have an impact on turning the situation around to a positive outcome. There are countless stories that document this occurrence, so when a newborn baby is lying in the neonatology department and fighting for life, or an older patient is in the Intensive Care Unit (ICU) and is struggling to stay alive, miracles do happen, and there is often no medical explanation for why they do. We just accept them with gratitude, and hope that the turnaround continues to full recovery. Medical miracles do happen. They do exist.

Our Story Continues
But let's get back to our discussion on birth to early adolescence, and let's first focus on the newborn who is fortunate to be born without a need for the intervention of a neonatologist. What are the reasonable expectations of the parents of the hospital, the doctors, the nurses, and the rest of the maternity and pediatric team?

Once the mother has gone into labor and the baby has been successfully delivered, the mother and her partner expect the hospital to keep the new mom comfortable, attend to her medical needs, and help her begin nursing and caring for her newborn child. Normal expectations that the new parents typically want met include that the hospital staff take good care of their child, that the nurses and doctors provide accurate information about any changing conditions in the health of the mother or the baby, that the hospital staff remain friendly and supportive, that the treatment plan as ordered by the OB/GYN be followed carefully, and that the entire hospital staff show compassion and interest in the newborn baby and the family.

Once the mother returns home, the next typical step is for the parents to select a pediatrician. Here again, there are many common reasonable expectations that parents have of the doctor and the staff in the doctor's office. Among them are the expectation that the pediatricians and their staff are friendly and kind to both the child and to the parents, that the providers and their staff respect the requests of the child, that the doctor reaches out to really get to know the child, that the doctor is constantly assessing physical, mental health, and emotional development of the child, that the doctor takes time to completely answer the questions of the child and the parents, and that the doctor strives at all times to gain the respect and trust of both the child who is the patient and the parents.

The Teen Years to Young Adulthood

Most children are followed by their pediatrician throughout their teen years until they reach college age, at which point most young adults choose to see a primary care physician and various specialists including an OB/GYN for women. When a child reaches their teen years, many of their expectations of their doctors change. One of the major changes is the reasonable expectation of confidentiality between the doctor and the patient. This issue has been discussed extensively. Much has been written about it. And so, as part of our exploration of patient centered care, we need to pause for a few moments, and look further into this issue.

Confidentiality and the Adolescent Patient

What exactly does healthcare law say about the rights of adolescent patients? Confidentiality in healthcare is extremely important to all patients of all ages. However, the line between what should stay confidential and what should not is blurry when it comes to teenagers. We know that parents and legal guardians are legally responsible for making the medical decisions of their children until the age of 18 years old. At the age of 18, in most states, a patient reaches the age of majority and has the right to make their own medical decisions. But the law gives thought to the needs and expectations of children, once they reach the age of 12 years old, although they are still legally minors.

It all comes down to the concept of *informed consent*. Informed consent is a healthcare law concept that obligates a physician to explain all of the details of any medical diagnosis or procedure including the risks, and at the same time, assess the patient's ability to make a medical decision. If the doctor believes that the patient has the capacity to make the decision for themselves and the patient signs the document called the informed consent form, the patient basically contracts with the doctor to do the procedure with the patient's full consent. Every state handles this issue differently. In New Jersey, a minor of 13 years or older can receive healthcare treatment or services without the need for a parent or guardian at a hospital, clinic, medical office or other facility when the concern deals with sexual assault, drug addiction or mental health services. These services are confidential so they are only dealt with between the patient and the physician, without getting a parent or guardian involved.

During their teen years, teens may undergo treatment or get checked out for concerns such as STDs, pregnancy, drug addiction or mental health, and wish that their information is kept confidential. Therefore, it has become important for a teenager to tell their physician about being sexually active, using drugs or any mental health concerns. This is crucial information that can impact the way the doctor treats the teen. Doctors assure their teen patients that they are not there to judge, only to ensure the safety in the treatment. The only instance where a provider will contact a parent or guardian is if behaviors can be dangerous to the teen's health, in which case it is the doctor's duty to inform the parent or legal guardian.

Another concern dealing with confidentiality for teens is payment. Teenagers often do not have the funds to be able to pay for such services and do not want to utilize insurance in fear that their parents or guardians will find out. It is suggested that they talk to the physician to see if they can stop the explanation of benefits billing or if there is an option to disable communication about healthcare services from the insurance agency to a parent or guardian. They can usually contact the insurance health plan and submit a Confidential Communications Request. This will ensure that parental figures will not be notified about healthcare services dealing with the topics of sex, drugs and mental health. These confidentiality protocols for teens are so important to allow them to utilize the healthcare services they need without worrying about their parents or guardians finding out. Insurance companies believe that just because teens are still minors, does not mean that they should not have access to the healthcare services that are crucial for their health, especially as they are growing.

The Age of Majority
When a child finally reaches the age of 18 years old, the young adult has full rights to self-determination. The patient makes their own medical decisions. At this point, if a person is going to college, often the medical staff at the college becomes the primary source of medical care. If the person is entering the military, the medical services of the service branch becomes the major source. If a person is not going to college or entering the military, and is going to work, most young adult patients find a primary care physician who will oversee their medical care, and will decide along with the patient, when it is appropriate to see a specialist, whether it be for gender health (urologist, OB/GYN), mental health, physical therapy or occupational therapy, eye care, or other specialists when required. According the Affordable Care Act, a patient may

remain on their parent's health insurance policy until they reach the age of 26 years old. However, if the young adult chooses not to, or they reach the age of 26, they then secure their own healthcare insurance, and typically if the insurance is not provided by their employer, they access the **Healthcare Marketplace**, which is another part of the Affordable Care Act to make insurance more affordable for an individual or young family.

In the next chapter, we will explore more about the reasonable expectations of the young adult.

Chapter Fifteen

Young Adult
By Anooshka Shukla

The patients in this demographic are ages 19 to 45. This group of patients may be the most resistant to going to see a doctor either because of lack of health insurance and/or they simply are healthier at this stage in life. I will examine patients of different genders and sexual orientation, races, socioeconomic status, religious practices, and level of education and explore how the Social Determinants of Health may differentiate patients from one another in the expectations they have. This is the stage in life when many of these patients start their careers, some marry, start a family, and decide where they wish to live, all important factors affecting their expectations as patients.

Introduction to the Young Adult Demographic
The young adult demographic is one of the largest demographics within the United States. As of 2019, there was an estimated 115,320 individuals between the ages of 19 to 45 (United States Bureau, 2021). This places a unique perspective on how the demographic is not only affected by the health conditions that can affect any demographic, such as diabetes and heart disease, but also in how they interact with the medical professionals such as doctors, nurses, therapists, and other healthcare workers. The young adult demographic experiences significant levels of different patient experiences that depend on their transitions from both adolescence to adulthood and young adult to middle age.

One aspect that defines the young adult demographic is their freedom to process, absorb, and obey the guidelines set by their doctor or trusted medical professional. How they decide to process this information is dependent on how their relationship is with their medical professional. Therefore, there is a bit of choice made on the patient's part for whether they wish either to comply with the guidelines of the provider or if they choose to continue with habits, routines, and lifestyles that can compromise their health. This aspect of the young adult demographic is affected by factors such as their previous patient experiences, their race/ethnicity, their socioeconomic status, gender, and level of education. These factors have significant influence on the health outcomes of the young adult demographic, affecting their physical health, mental health, and emotional health.

Reasonable Expectations of the Patient
The expectations of the patient of the medical provider play a significant role in health outcome and status. But what exactly are the expectations that a young adult patient has of their medical provider, if they have the goal of getting the best patient centered care possible? One of the most important factors is approachability and friendliness, so that the provider can fully empathize and know what the patient has experienced. Another important reasonable expectation is *confidentiality*, so the young adult patient can be assured that what they share with their doctor remains private. The third major expectation is that the provider will work with the patient in terms of affording treatment and medication, since many individuals in this patient population have just completed their undergraduate or graduate education, are saddled with student debt, may be just starting their career in an entry level job, or recently married and perhaps starting a family. So, typically the young adult expects guidance and understanding from their provider to help the patient navigate the healthcare delivery system in the most cost-effective way possible without compromising good health care.

The young adult patient tends to shy away from using the healthcare system unless there is an urgent reason to visit a doctor or a hospital. Again, this is due to several factors – the cost of seeing a doctor and paying out of pocket, the high cost of buying healthcare insurance, the belief of many young adults that they are strong and healthy, even when they are not, and not making the time to schedule routine exams and immunizations, choosing instead to spend their money and using their time to work out at the gym with the goal of staying healthy. For this reason, unfortunately, many serious healthcare conditions particular to the young adult patient population go undiagnosed until it becomes too late to reverse the condition. Of course, this becomes even a greater problem when the patient is low-income or living far away from decent healthcare or is lacking the education to realize the value of maintaining their health.

Chapter Sixteen

Middle Age
By Abigail Arient

When patients reach middle age, they begin a new journey in terms of their health. Potentially encountering conditions that many of these patients will have to face and cope with for the rest of their lives, patient centered care for middle aged patients is very much expected. This second to last stage of life is one that can often be skipped over or ignored and this plays a part in the treatment of middle aged patients.

Middle Age is the time of life beyond young adulthood and before old age. People identified as middle aged are between the ages of 45-65 years old, and this is the phase in life when many people start to encounter health problems related to aging.

We have all heard stories about mid-life crisis. It is a real psychological phenomena that often occurs during middle age where one experiences concerns about their identity, their self-confidence, and their life choices. This phenomenon occurs often as one first noticeable signs of aging either physically and/or mentally. It is often the first time a person needs to accept that they are getting older and that aging is simply a part of life.

Very often, men experience what has been called *andropause*. Andropause is a syndrome of aging that is associated with decrease in libido, low testosterone levels, and an overall decrease in general well being. It is also referred to as "male menopause." This is one way to describe and term the hormonal and reproductive changes experienced by middle aged men due to aging.

At the same time, middle age is when women experience *menopause*, which is the natural process undergone by women between the ages of 45-55 in which the ovaries cease hormone production. As a result of the decrease in reproductive hormones, menopause arrives twelve months after the last date of a woman's period. Broken down into three stages, premenopause, menopause, and post menopause, each stage has different symptoms. Again, it is a common signal for women that the body is changing and the woman is growing older. For this reason, many women need to turn to support groups to get through this stage, which can be very uncomfortable both physically and emotionally. Symptoms of menopause include irregular periods, fatigue, mood swings, insomnia, hot flashes, night sweats, loss of libido and sexual discomfort. Other symptoms include anxiety and depression, for many women menopause is physiological reminder of their advancement in age with the end of their child-bearing years. Treatments are all focused on symptomatic relief and come in many different forms which are necessary to adapt and meet the needs of patient preferences and allergies to certain medications. These various treatments for menopause include oral hormone therapies, estrogens, dietary supplements, and topical lubricants. With such distinct transitions in reproductive health for middle aged patients, this area of treatment is unique to this population.

Some Other New Healthcare Experiences
Middle aged patients start to see more obvious signs of aging that can both be visible cosmetically as well as less visible in terms of cognitive signs of aging. Middle aged patients must cope with these new signs and symptoms of aging and have special treatment aimed for their population as well. For example, recommended regular colonoscopies start for middle aged patients at age 50 with routine check ups every 1 to 3 years as recommended by the American Cancer Society. Women also begin to have mammograms annually at this stage of their lives. Patients may also need to start routine visits to certain specialists like cardiologists, endocrinologists,

ENT physicians and audiologists to examine hearing loss, rheumatologists for diseases like arthritis and back pain, and orthopedists, who the patient may need to see for sports injuries or joint replacements.

At the same time, middle aged patients, both men and women, also encounter changes in reproductive health. For men, erectile dysfunction (ED) is a common condition that is encountered by about thirty million men in the United States alone, according to the National Institute of Diabetes and Digestive Kidney Disease. While ED can happen to any man regardless of age, it is more common in older men. The average age range for the onset of ED is between the ages of 40 and 70. It is important to communicate any ED symptoms with a healthcare provider as it could be a sign of a more serious health problem or concern, especially heart disease.

How are Middle Age Patients Treated as Patients?
The middle age period of life is much more than just an age range and set time in the overall human lifespan. Middle aged patients need to face physiological, psychological, and social issues at this time in life. Often it is a time when people look back on their accomplishments, vocational or otherwise, and look forward to facing a future that some have been running from while others have embraced. Such an important transitional period, bridging young adulthood to old age, is one that is often looked over, and providing patient centered care and meeting the reasonable expectations of these patients is most important to this patient population.

Middle aged patients face a societal and stereotypical challenge of "the mid-life crisis." This phenomenon's impact on patient centered care and healthcare in general is one that has a direct influence on how middle aged patients are viewed and treated. Patients often complain about not being taken seriously when concerns or complications are brought up. A mid-life crisis is an easy explanation for the many changes, health related or otherwise, that middle aged patients may experience during this period of their lives. Another common complaint is that middle aged patients feel stuck in terms of their healthcare and treatment. All these sentiments and more are captured best through the patient stories below.

Patient Stories
Terry is a 49 year old patient that feels stuck in his path of healthcare and treatment options. Enjoying a life of good health and days filled with activity, this all changed on one evening. Terry survived a bad car accident at the age of 44. While lucky and grateful to have survived, he did not come out unscathed. Terry had suffered herniated discs in his back as a result of the accident and ever since has never been the same. Activities he once enjoyed like jogging, hiking, and going on roller coasters with his family now come with sudden aches and pains that last for days. Even everyday activities such as putting on shoes are now more difficult than before. When he visited the doctor for possible advice and hopeful treatment, he was left with a disappointing answer. He was told that he was too young for the back surgery that was recommended for such injuries and was not given other options than cortisone injections. Terry says that his pain has not been taken seriously and each time he goes back to the doctor his pains are blamed on other health problems. He has been told to "just lose weight" and then all the issues he is dealing with will get better. However, following the accident, exercising now hurts more than ever. Terry now finds himself stuck waiting for eventual back surgery coping with the pain in the meantime.

Stephanie is a 47 year old mother of two and an office manager. Stephanie was recently diagnosed as pre-diabetic for Type 2 diabetes following her annual visit with her primary care provider. This means that without intervention mainly in the form of lifestyle changes, Stephanie is at risk of developing diabetes within the next ten years. Eager to reverse and try to prevent that from happening Stephanie has tried to develop a plan to do so. Stephanie feels that other than the diagnosis, her provider has not given much help or assistance in how to approach preventing the onset of the disease, other than changing her medications. Without much of a care plan, Stephanie has turned to friends and family members for advice. Having a more structured plan of action from her provider would make Stephanie feel better about tackling these new lifestyle changes in order to ensure that she will not need daily insulin injections for the rest of her life. While motivated to make changes, Stephanie feels stuck and unsure where to start.

Reasonable Expectations of Patients
As seen through the patient stories, there are expectations of middle aged patients that are often not met. These expectations are reasonable, but providers respond that the symptoms can be attributed to aging. Patients expect to receive methods of treatment and approaches to care that align with patient centered care. However, when the patient centered care approach is not always implemented in all healthcare settings, it leaves many patients stuck and frustrated. As such, this can alienate or push patients away and discourage them from seeking medical care due to prior frustrating situations in regards to insurance, quality of care, or availability of practitioners.

Middle aged patients can often feel brushed aside or ignored when facing the onset of new health concerns. As such, many patients find themselves putting off care until they are eligible for Medicare after turning 65. Many middle aged patients believe that when they begin receiving Medicare, it will open the doors to options that are not yet available to them. This can be detrimental to patient health as waiting could make a problem or condition that could have been addressed sooner, worse in the long run. While wanting to wait for more affordable and comprehensive care that is available later in life works for some, this should not have to be the reality and solution that every middle aged patient faces.

Middle aged patients have reasonable expectations of receiving care and help in their transition from adulthood into later geriatric stages of life and for many, during their middle ages is the first time they are encountering health issues and complications.

Solutions
While it may seem obvious that the solution to these issues is the proper implementation of patented centered care, that is easier said than done. Focusing on the individual when it comes to treatment and care is a pivotal way to start. Making sure the patient feels involved through education and understanding can transform the patient care process. The middle aged patient wants to be heard and wants to be believed. They want compassion from their providers as they experience the health related transitions that begin at this point in life and become even more pronounced as the reach their final stage in their healthcare journey, becoming a senior patient.

Allowing middle-aged patients to properly express concerns and help them work towards solutions and make plans of actions to address any issues is one main way that a provider can approach middle aged patients through the lens of patient centered care. Recognizing how middle age is so much more than just a chronological age and implementing this mentality to practice and treatment is a way to establish a relationship of patient centered care towards middle aged patients. While simply listening and talking to a patient does not seem like the most groundbreaking solution, it is one that creates a space through approaches of patient centered care that allows middle aged patients to feel comfortable in seeking help and expressing concerns when it comes to their changing health needs and the impacts of aging. Making sure that patients do not feel alone or alienated provides support that can help one cope with the changes in lifestyle and health. Acknowledging the multidimensionality of middle aged patients and responding to their expectations as patients is essential to patient centered care.

Chapter Seventeen

Senior Years
By Dima Bischoff-Hashem and Anat Ferleger

This chapter will focus on the level of patient centered care that a patient expects and receives in their senior years, from age 61 years old to 95 years old. Using interviews and literature to examine how senior citizens are treated as patients, this chapter will examine the common expectations of this population and how providers respond to those expectations.

Medicare

When a person reaches the age of 65, something wonderful happens in their lifelong healthcare journey. They become eligible for Medicare, a federal program that provides healthcare coverage to all seniors throughout the United States who qualify. For most individuals, it is something they look forward to as they reach older age.

You become qualified for Medicare if you are over the age of 65, and are either a United States citizen or a permanent legal resident. If one suffers from End-Stage Renal Disease or ALS, they are may apply earlier for coverage, as well as those who are under the age of 65 who are deemed medically disabled and have received 24 consecutive months of disability payments from Social Security. For most Americans, individuals may apply three months before they turn 65.

The Medicare program is divided into four parts. Medicare *Part A* is known as the original Medicare. It is free for all individuals who have personally or who are married to someone who has paid their Medicare taxes for at least ten years. If you are not eligible for free coverage, you are able to pay a monthly premium to acquire coverage. Medicare Part A covers the cost of inpatient hospital care, skilled nursing facility admissions, hospice, and home health care. *Part B* provides coverage for doctors' visits, mental health care, medical equipment, physical and occupational therapy, diagnostic testing, some cancer treatments as well as preventative health care services. Some preventative health care services covered include one's annual wellness visit, colorectal cancer screenings, cardiovascular disease screenings and specific vaccinations. The cost of Medicare Part B varies depending on one's annual income, but does not cover 100 percent of expenses. Individuals are still responsible for covering what Medicare does not pay for. *Part D* is available to help cover the cost of prescription drugs. All plans are required to cover medications in specific categories, such as cancer medications and those used to treat HIV. However, each plan is formatted in a different way and the cost varies dramatically from plan to plan.

Because Medicare does not pay the whole bill, individuals with traditional Medicare are given the option of adding a separate plan, known as *Medigap* to help cover expenses such as copayments, coinsurance, deductibles, and other expenses. This coverage is highly recommended. It comes at an additional monthly cost. It is offered by many private insurance companies. Medigap policies are identified with the letters A through F, all offering the different benefits, and the more benefits that the Medigap plan has, the greater the cost for the patient. If one can acquire supplemental insurance through an employer or union instead of a Medigap plan, that is usually recommended.

Another option is the Medicare Advantage plan, which is an alternative to signing up for the original Medicare. It is often known as *Part C*, however once enrolled you are no longer a part of original Medicare. It is offered through many private insurance companies. It is generally less expensive, since most patients on the original Medicare plan tend to sign up for additional coverage, as well as the Medigap plan. Prescription medications, as well as an over-the-counter drug allowance are also included in the Medicare Advantage plan, as well as all other services covered in Parts A and D of the original Medicare, but not Part B. Vision care, hearing, and dental services, as well as some transport services are also covered with fewer restrictions. Patients are also responsible for covering their copays and coinsurance. Other costs include monthly premiums, and deductibles for medical services, as well as for drug coverage. Many patients opt for a Medicare Advantage plan since they contract to only pay a fixed amount of out of pocket for medical services.

For those who qualify for Medicare, but cannot afford the out of pocket portion, there is the *Medicare Savings Program*, which is available to low-income seniors and patients with disabilities to help with the financial cost of health care. This program helps users cover the cost of premiums, deductibles, coinsurances, and copayments. However only those who financially qualify receive this assistance.

Common Health Issues That Senior-Aged Patients Face
There are a variety of health issues seniors face as their bodies begin to age. Nevertheless, according to the CDC, 40% of adults age 65 and older report being in good or excellent health. With the life expectancy in the United States continuing to rise, it is projected that this percentage will become higher. Regardless of how a senior patient feels, it is essential that seniors are aware of common health issues that may arise so they can stay ahead of the issues and take care of their health.

While lifestyle plays a vital role in one's health, one's genetics, age and family history play a large factor in one's risk for developing certain conditions. Listed below are the most commonly reported issues in adults 65 years and up and ways to help lower one's risk of disease.

Heart Disease
Heart disease is the leading cause of death in adults 65 and older. According to the CDC, 21.7% of adults ages 65 and older report being diagnosed with coronary heart disease (CHD) and/or stroke. The prevalence of CHD and/or stroke is higher among men than women. Data from the CDC shows that the prevalence also varies among racial/ethnic groups: 14.8% of whites, 14.9% of blacks/African Americans, 11.2% of Hispanics, and 8.2% of Asians and Pacific Islanders. One is also twice as likely to develop CHD and/or stroke if they have less than high school education compared to those with a post high school education. According to heart.org, 80% of cardiovascular diseases, including those discussed above are preventable. Some things you can do to help prevent the development of heart disease are to maintain a healthy weight, exercise, quit smoking if you do, avoid excess amounts of alcohol, develop strategies to manage stress, and maintain healthy cholesterol levels.

Cognitive Decline
Mild memory loss is common as one ages. However the development of Alzheimer's Disease is not. According to the CDC, 1 in 9 people ages 65 and older have Alzheimer's Disease, which is a disease of the brain that slowly compromises a person's memory and body functions. While you cannot prevent the development of Alzheimer's Disease, it is essential to recognize early symptoms as early intervention is key to help slow the progression of the disease. Therefore, the
Centers for Medicare and Medicaid Services, which oversees the Medicare and Medicaid programs, mandates that patients over 65 have a short memory test when they are given their annual wellness exam by their primary care physician. The allows the PCP to detect early memory loss and refer the patient to a neurologist, if necessary.

Balance issues
Falls are a leading cause of injury in seniors. According to the CDC, more than one in four adults fall each year. In 2020,

36,507 seniors ages 65 and older died from preventable falls, while 2.8 million were treated in an emergency department. According to health.gov, some ways to reduce the likelihood of falls are by adapting one's home to make it safer and more accessible, exercising regularly, looking over medication side effects, and being aware of hearing and vision changes, and addressing them.

Oral health problems
Oral health issues are also common in seniors. Specifically gingivitis, which can lead to periodontitis. This is a bacterial infection which can affect the health of one's gums and bones. The CDC estimates that 2 in 3 adults ages 65 and older have gum disease in the United States. Maintaining proper oral care, as well as seeing a dentist every six months is the best way to help prevent oral health issues from arising.

Osteoarthritis and Osteoporosis
Osteoporosis is defined as a disease in which one's bones weaken to the point where they break easily. It progresses slowly over time and one usually does not notice any changes until they begin to break bones. It is estimated that 54 million adults over the age of 50 have low bone mass and/or osteoporosis. Osteoarthritis is the most common form of arthritis and according to the National Osteoporosis Foundation, almost all adults over the age of 80 have some form of it. Although it is not entirely preventable, exercising regularly and eating a healthy diet can help keep your bones and joints protected.

Respiratory Diseases
Adults are at risk for a whole host of respiratory diseases. Conditions such as asthma and chronic obstructive pulmonary disease usually worsen as one ages. It is estimated that around 1 in 7, 15% of adults in the United States suffer from one or more lung diseases. According to a medical advisor to the American Lung Association "There are a huge number of

Americans that experience lung obstruction". It is the third leading cause of death in the United States. Not smoking, or stopping as soon as possible if you do smoke is a major way to reduce your risk of developing a respiratory disease. Exercising, being up to date on vaccines and screening are other actions you can take to help protect your lungs.

Vision and Hearing Loss
Age related eye issues, such as macular degeneration, cataracts and glaucoma are a growing issue that affect millions of seniors. As for hearing, 43% of people over 65 and older experience some form of hearing loss. Maintaining regular screenings for both hearing and vision is essential for all adults. Protecting one's eye from the sun can help reduce vision deterioration. Avoiding constant and loud noises can also help protect one's hearing and reduce hearing loss.

What Issues Do Seniors Face in Accessing Patient-Centered Care?
Senior-age patients face a host of issues accessing quality patient-centered care. Some of the most significant hurdles, and the ones we will discuss, are finding doctors who accept Medicare, receiving care for health problems not covered by Medicare, and traveling to appointments.

Finding a Doctor Who Accepts Medicare
Arguably, finding a doctor who accepts Medicare is the biggest difficulty senior-age patients face in accessing health care. The Healthcare Leadership Council states that 83 percent of doctors accepted Medicare patients in 2010; now that number has gone down to 81 percent. One reason providers are increasingly turning down Medicare patients is that they have to file extensive paperwork for the patients to get coverage. If providers fill out paperwork incorrectly, or don't follow the Medicare standard of care exactly, they could be required to return some of the Medicare payments and possibly be sued.

Therefore, it is less profitable and more time consuming for healthcare providers to accept Medicare than private insurance. Additionally, while Medicare pays physicians a percentage of their posted fees, on average private insurance pays physicians 143 percent of Medicare rates according to Kaiser Family Foundation. People in rural areas can have a particular difficulty finding physicians that accept Medicare because there are already fewer physicians in those areas.

Not Everything is Covered
Long-term custodial care, most dental care, eye exams, hearing aids and exams, and most foot care are not included in Medicare coverage. Therefore, senior age patients must pay out of pocket for these treatments and services. According to the Administration for Community Living, 65 year-olds today have a seventy percent chance of needing long-term care before they pass away. In some situations, family members and friends can take on a caretaker role. However, for an individual working full time, caring for children, or living far away from their elderly relative, placing their relative in a nursing home or paying for in-home care are often the only options. Depending on the state and whether the senior's room is semi-private or private, the monthly cost for a nursing home ranges from $6,000 to $15,000 dollars (excluding Alaska where it costs over $30,000 dollars). According to CNBC, the median 401(k) balance of people 65 or older is $82,000 dollars. That means spending one year in a nursing home would drain the average person's retirement savings. Adding to that, dental care, eye exams, hearing aids, and foot care, since they are not covered by Medicare, also consume a person's retirement savings. For example, over 90 percent of Medicare recipients age 65 and older report wearing glasses, yet they have to pay out of pocket for prescriptions.

Traveling to Doctor's Appointments
Many elderly patients have trouble physically getting to doctor's appointments. In fact, driving short distances and

walking even from the parking lot to the waiting room can be a difficult task. According to the Pierre Paul Driving School in Brooklyn, New York, drivers over age 75 cause more accidents than middle aged drivers. One reason could be, 80 percent of people in their 70s have arthritis restricting movement and making it more difficult to grip the steering wheel. Older drivers are also more fragile and have slower reaction times, making observing other vehicles, turning, and breaking in time more difficult, and meaning accidents are more likely to be fatal. Therefore, asking an elderly patient to drive to appointments puts them and other drivers at risk. Public transportation is a reliable alternative to driving in some major cities, but for the most part, it is sparse and poorly-funded throughout the United States, and many seniors have a hard time waiting for the bus and/or boarding it because of mobility or cognitive issues. Additionally, house calls, which made up forty percent of all doctors' appointments in the 1940s, have now become almost obsolete.

How Do the Social Determinants of Health Affect Senior Care?
By looking at the Social Determinants of Health, we can understand the various experiences senior patients experience based on *economic stability, social and community context, neighborhood, and built environment*, and other factors. In the above section, we briefly discussed the ways economic stability can impact senior patients' access to healthcare. Less financially stable seniors may not be able to afford eye exams, hearing aids, dental care, and other healthcare not covered by Medicare. Long-term care, which may be necessary for some elderly people, is also unaffordable for many and is also not covered by Medicare. Additionally, commuting to a doctor can be a taxing and dangerous task for senior patients' whose impaired vision and slow reflexes inhibit their driving. Those with the money to do so can pay for taxis or ride services. Ultimately, difficulty accessing all these types of care means financially unstable seniors are relegated to spend their final years living a poor quality of life. That is, unless they have a

network of devoted and close by family members or friends to take care of them. This is where social and community context comes in. If elderly people have friends or family to drive them to appointments and help them cook and clean, they can live more comfortably through their senior years. Finally, aspects of built environment, such as access to public transportation and proximity to doctor's offices strongly impact the ability to obtain health care for seniors.

Improving Seniors' Experiences at the Doctors

So, how can we as a society improve the experiences of seniors accessing patient-centered care? While many of the necessary changes are systemic and require policy changes, medical staff and seniors can both take actions to improve the experiences of senior patients. To start, physicians' offices can explain what Medicare covers to their senior patients. According to data journalist Dan Grunebaum, a quarter of those enrolled in Medicare don't understand their plans well. Additionally, since many seniors have limited access to transportation and might have specific days when they can travel to appointments with their doctors, front desk staff can prioritize appointment times for seniors. Physician office staff can also make accommodations for seniors related to inclement weather. For example if the ground is snowy or icy, staff can walk seniors to and from their cars.

Along those lines, seniors who take taxis often end up standing outside large medical buildings waiting for their ride to pick them up. Office staff can help with this by calling taxis for seniors and walking them to the taxi. Slowing down and having patience on the phone and in the office when talking with seniors can create a safer, more comforting environment, more conducive to seniors sharing their issues and asking for what they need. Finally, employing social workers as part of a patient care team in the office can improve the senior patient experience. Trained social workers can have slower conversations with seniors, get to know their needs and set up outside services.

Chapter Eighteen

End of Life
By Bob Kieserman

This is the final chapter of this section we have called Life Cycles, where we looked at the expectations of the parents of the very youngest patients up to the very oldest patients. While chronologically it seems appropriate that when discussing the end of life, we should focus on the senior population, unfortunately, we all know that end of life can sadly happen at any time during a lifetime. And so, for the sake of exploring how patient centered care is so important at this point in life, this chapter will focus on the experiences and expectations of a patient at any age to explain this final part of the life cycle.

When someone has lived their life and that life is coming to an end and the patient only has a few months, weeks, days, or hours to live, they understandably have many reasonable expectations. Perhaps more than at any other time in their life. When someone learns that they are terminally ill, it is not only a great shock and life changing, but a patient begins to brainstorm with the help of doctors and family members what possible next steps can be taken to prolong life as long as possible through the wonderful advancements in medicine we are so privileged to have. It is normal for a patient to become focused on expectations; expectations of the providers, expectations of the healthcare facilities, expectations of the health insurance company, expectations of family, and expectations of others who will influence the patient's care.

In order to explore how patient centered care is provided at the end of life, it is first important to define some essential terms for our discussion.

DEFINITIONS

END OF LIFE: When providers and patients define the term end of life, they are referring to the point where a patient, due to a sudden or a prolonged medical situation, is facing a prognosis of death in a period of hours, days, weeks, months, or within a year.

THE RIGHT OF SELF-DETERMINATION: When a patient faces that prognosis, the patient's right of self-determination becomes very important. The right to self-determination, discussed earlier in the book, is defined as a patient's legal right to decide whether they agree to medical treatment including hospitalization, procedures, surgery, treatment plans, and taking prescribed medication. According to the National Library of Medicine, this right is protected by **The Patient Self-Determination Act** (PSDA), a federal law making compliance mandatory. The purpose of this act to ensure that a patient's right to self-determination in health care decisions be communicated and protected. Through advance directives--the living will and the durable power of attorney--the right to accept or reject medical or surgical treatment is available to adults while competent, so that in the event that such adults become incompetent to make decisions, they would more easily continue to control decisions affecting their health care through declared instructions to their family and to the medical team.

THE FIDUCIARY RELATIONSHIP AND DURABLE POWER OF ATTORNEY: When a patient is no longer able to make their own medical decision, by having drafted a *Living Will* or *Advance Directive* with an attorney while they were alert and competent, a named surrogate decision maker, normally a spouse or adult child, is granted the legal right to make sure that the parameters the patient made in the Living Will or Advance Directive, are carried out completely in terms of medical care.

CAPACITY: When providers are deciding a treatment plan for a patient, it is the provider's obligation to fully explain to the patient the benefits and the risks of the plan, and to get the patient's legal consent. This consent is called Informed Consent. However, there are times, especially at the end of life, when a provider needs to determine whether the patient has the cognitive ability to understand what is being explained by the provider. This is known as capacity. According to research conducted by Hugo Amador, one of my co-authors, it is common that in certain medical situations, many patients cannot make their own medical decisions pertaining to their illness or overall health. This is what is called having lost *decisional capacity*. Around 40% of medical inpatients and residential hospice patients reach decisional incapacity and roughly 90% of adults reach decisional incapacity in intensive care units.

Providers and physicians intuitively assess capacity based on four elements: understanding what is being said to the patient, appreciation for what is being said, reasoning and the ability to weigh the options, and communication, the ability to have a dialogue with the medical staff. Should a patient's dialogue not proceed in a logical fashion, then the provider seeks alternate means for the patient's decision making.

Hugo Amador further explains that in terms of informed consent, the provider is obligated to educate the patient about the risks, benefits, and alternatives of a proposed treatment or intervention. The patient must be competent enough in order to make a voluntary decision. The Joint Commission requires documentation of all elements of informed consent which include (1) the nature of the procedure; (2) the risks and benefits of the procedure; (3) reasonable alternatives; (4) risks and benefits of the alternatives; and (5) an assessment of the patient's understanding of elements (1) through (4). It is important that the provider avoid making the patient feel forced to agree with the provider and thus must only make a recommendation and provide reasoning for said recommendation.

What Are the Reasonable Expectations of the Patient?
Regardless of the age or gender or ethnic background of the patient, all patients expect undivided attention from the healthcare team when they are hospitalized. This is especially true at the end of life. Because each second literally counts, patients expect that doctors, nurses, therapists, and technicians will be mindful of the patient's fragile condition, and providing a comfortable hospital room, quality care, complete disclosure by the healthcare team of the constantly changing treatment plan, adherence by the medical staff to the conditions set by the patient in their Advance Directive, and honoring the patient's right to make decisions about their care as long as the patient is conscious and capable of making decisions.

What Are the Reasonable Expectations of the Family?
Typically, the patient themselves or through the directions of the Advance Directive, gives permission to the healthcare providers to share updates about the patient's condition with family. Therefore, if this permission has been established, the family expects full disclosure by the medical team on the patient's prognosis, updates on the patient's condition, and clear and honest communication of the treatment options. The family also expects respect for the family by the healthcare team as well as compassion for those who eventually become the surrogate decision makers making important decisions for the patient. Finally, the family expects accommodations by the hospital and medical staff for the mental and physical wellbeing of the family to help the family cope with the stress and anxiety that watching a loved one die brings.

When patients and their families have been asked about their expectations at the end of life, patients and families emphasize the importance of health personnel anticipating illness changes and recognizing the information and palliation required to keep the patient comfortable. Family members who became proxy decision-makers have reported uncertainty and distress when guidance from health personnel is lacking. Families worry about staff shortages and emphasize how important it is to them that the doctors be available and accessible. Relatives and health personnel seldom respect the ability of an aware patient to consent to their own treatment, and too often the preferences of the patient are not always recognized.

Do Expectations Differ Based on The Social Determinants of Health?

With that said, I want to focus on six of the Social Determinants of Health – education of the patient, community and social context, gender of the patient, age of the patient, the economic stability of the patient, and the patient's access to healthcare - in exploring patent centered care at the end of the life. All of these Social Determinants of Health were defined and discussed in Chapter Two. How do these variables affect the patient's perception of care at the end of a patient's life and why is that important?

The Education of the Patient

It would make sense that the more educated a patient and/or the patient's family is about what is reasonable to expect when a patient is hospitalized at the end of life, the more the patient and/or the family can advocate for the best patient centered care possible. Those patients and family members who have the education and experiences that make them a better consumer of healthcare typically receive more attention and even better care at this final stage of life. We know that there are ethnic groups and cultures who, through a history of one generation teaching another, have great fears of being hospitalized and an underlying mistrust for doctors and medicine, in general. In a 2020 article for the American

Medical Student Association, Shruthi Reddy asserted the factors that impact cultural and educational differences in embracing healthcare experiences "include family roles, body language, concept of justice, notions of modesty, core values, family values, beliefs and assumptions, rules of conduct, expectations, gestures, and childrearing practices, all of which have been shown to influence our perception and approaches to health and medicine". It has also been determined by leading medical sociologists that patients with less formal education tend to either shy away from going to a hospital or once they enter a hospital, most likely through the emergency room, either surrender themselves to whatever it being performed on them without question, or they show distrust for every medical intervention that the medical staff is trying to offer, often making themselves difficult patients to treat.

The Community and Social Context of the Patient

Patients who are at the end of their life need to feel embraced and supported by their family, friends, and neighbors. Studies have shown that patients who are not alone in the hospital, or at home surrounded by others close to them, die more peacefully when they know their family is with them. This became very evident when protocols enacted by hospitals throughout the country prevented family members from being with their loved ones during the COVID-19 hospitalizations, and many patients sadly died from the disease alone in their hospital bed. This put great strain on both the patients and on their families and friends. Many patients, whether very religious or not, also benefit from knowing that their religious congregations, family, and friends, are praying for their recovery, and this is especially important in many ethnic groups and cultures that are faith focused. With the advent of social media, many end of life patients also receive much comfort receiving messages and posts from family, friends, and also supportive strangers virtually on such sites as Facebook, Linkedin, and Twitter. People need to feel connected, and this is especially true when a patient is facing the end of life. Support of the community and social contacts are most important to the healing of the patient and the patient's will to live.

The Gender of the Patient

As we learned earlier in Chapter Eight, medical sociologists have identified the fact that women tend to be more proactive patients than men. While women tend to address concerns about their health, men typically wait until the pain or the seriousness of their ailment is too great to tolerate and then they decide to seek medical attention. Therefore, research has told us that men tend to be more passive at the end of life, and the responsibility of advocating for patient centered care falls on family and friends. Likewise, because end of life can occur at any time in a person's lifetime, often even younger men need to be convinced and encouraged by their doctors, family, and friends to take more aggressive measures to prolong their life, especially when faced with a terminal condition. Women need less encouragement, and tend to be more open to and more proactive to seeking life prolonging measures.

In terms of who receives better patient centered care, there is no indication that it depends so much on gender, but rather on the patient's ability and willingness to make medical decisions and/or the support system that the patient has. It is true that the argument has been made that male healthcare providers sometimes carry a bias against female patients, with female providers being more compassionate and more responsive to both women and men as their patients. The research seems to support this including a study that MedFocus Research conducted in 2021 where it was found that women physicians showed more understanding for the patient's needs than male physicians. However, at the end of life, because of the literal life and death situation that providers and medical support staff are facing on an hour to hour basis, the bias, if it exists, is often overlooked by the patient, because perhaps at no other time in a patient's life, is a patient more dependent on those taking care of them, and keeping the patient comfortable takes priority.

At the same time, much has been written and researched about the attitude of healthcare providers on the patients from the LGBTQ+ community. Research has proven that there are many health disparities for this patient population as discussed earlier in the book in Chapter 13 on Access to Healthcare, even at the very end of life. And so, at the end of their life, many members of this community may claim not to receive the same attention and treatment that others in the overall patient community receive. This has been documented, and this is most disturbing. Certainly it is one of the greatest concerns of the medical community right now and a high priority of medical schools and residency programs. Through new initiatives, new doctors are learning to be more open to the lifestyles and special medical needs of the LGBTQ+ patient community, especially at the end of life, and to improve the care that the LGBTQ+ patient receives.

The Age of the Patient
Of all of the Social Determinants of Health that impact patient centered care at the end of life, probably the most relevant is the age of the patient. None of us know when the end of our life will occur. While we hope we live a long life, sadly that does not always happen. Many studies have been done on how age affects how a patient is treated at the end of life, and medical sociologists have found that of all patient populations, older patients over the age of 80 are the group that has the most differences in terms of patient care at the end of life. The

biggest difference is that younger patients typically are able to face their medical condition with clarity and full understanding of treatment options, while the care of seniors may be complicated by age-related dementia and an overall slowing of their cognitive abilities.

We also know that while there are exceptions. The older a patient becomes, typically the more a patient interacts with the healthcare delivery system. And so, as a person becomes older, at each stage of their life, they gain more experience with illnesses, treatments, options, and interactions with healthcare providers. To a child who is very ill, it is very frightening, and they need to put trust in their parents and in the healthcare providers. That is why the doctors and support staff at our children's hospitals deserve our greatest appreciation for the wonderful work they do. To a college student who learns that they have cancer, it is also usually a new experience, especially if they have been healthy up until then. But because a college student has had some interaction with healthcare providers as a child and a teenager, they are usually able to be a more responsive patient and handle the news of the diagnosis with more clarity and objectivity. To a middle-aged patient, since they have already lived half their life, although dealing with terminal illness is difficult, again, they can face it with some experience and objectivity. When a person reaches old age, and they are now facing the end of their life, there is often more acceptance of what is happening, but nevertheless, there is sadness, concern for loved ones, and a need to make sure that their family members will be all right after they pass.

There are those who say that age affects the way a patient is treated. That is why a patient being treated for a terminal disease benefits from having a doctor who specializes not only in the illness, but the age group, as well. For example, children who are very ill, benefit more by being in a children's hospital, rather than a general hospital. In the children's hospital, the doctors and the entire support staff are focused on pediatric care. Likewise, when an older patient becomes ill, they will benefit more by being treated by specialists who focus on geriatric care, who understand the needs of older patients as well as their personal and medical expectations.

The Economic Stability of the Patient

Perhaps one of the biggest worries that a dying patient has is that the care they are receiving is very expensive and their families are going to be burdened with the bill. Most patients at the end of life hope that their medical insurance pays for the intensive care they are receiving, but at the back of a patient's mind, is what if the insurance does not cover some of this, will I be leaving my family with a huge debt. That is why the economic stability of the patient is a key factor in the sociological considerations of end of life. If a patient has been fortunate to put away money throughout their life to support unforeseen situations like a sudden illness, the patient lies in the hospital bed with less worry and concern. If, however, the patient has not been able to create an economic reserve throughout their life, regardless of how long that life has been, this insecurity can weigh heavily on the patient as they lie in the hospital bed, and this great concern can often compromise the patient's ability to fight for life. Economic concerns are stressful for any person of any age, but to be facing death and knowing that your family may be saddled with enormous debt because of the very expensive end of life medical interventions that are being performed on you, can be devastating to a patient's peace and comfort at the end of their life. This is especially true if the patient has no secondary medical insurance, and the family is depending on Medicare, Medicaid, or charity to pay the treatment the patient is receiving. The patient may have been unemployed at the time of the health crisis, or underemployed, or even living in poverty. As we will see in the next section on access to care, the hospital will still admit the patient, but how the bill will be paid remains the concern for many patients.

Access of Healthcare at the End of Life

Healthcare law in the United States mandates that any patient who is admitted to a hospital that accepts Medicare payments, which almost all hospitals do, must be treated and cared for, regardless of whether they have medical insurance. According to archives of the United States Congress, "The Emergency Medical Treatment and Active Labor Act (EMTALA) was passed by Congress in 1986 as part of the Consolidated Omnibus Reconciliation Act (COBRA), much of which dealt with Medicare issues. The law's initial intent was to ensure patient access to emergency medical care and to prevent the practice of patient dumping, in which uninsured patients were transferred, solely for financial reasons, from private to public hospitals without consideration of their medical condition or stability for the transfer. Although only 4 pages in length and barely noticed at the time, EMTALA has created a storm of controversy over the ensuing 15 years, and it is now considered one of the most comprehensive laws guaranteeing nondiscriminatory access to emergency medical care and thus to the health care system. Even though its initial language covered the care of emergency medical conditions, through interpretations by the Health Care Financing Administration (HCFA) (now known as the Centers for Medicare and Medicaid Services), the agency that oversees EMTALA enforcement, as well as various court decisions, the statute now potentially applies to virtually all aspects of patient care in the hospital setting."

And so, as a result, many hospitals in lower income neighborhoods admit hundreds of patients a month without insurance, and they must give them the same quality of care as they would to a patient with insurance. For an older patient, the hospital can bill Medicare. However, for a patient younger

than 65 years old, the hospital may be spending tens of thousands of dollars in treating that patient at the end of their life with no possible way to get compensated, other than
passing the costs on to the family of the patient. So, I guess if there is any positive aspect to a dying person's access to healthcare, the right to be admitted to a hospital and be treated, is it. However, the debt that the hospitalization may create for the patient's family is the unfortunate flip side of this situation. In reality, many hospitals are not able to collect the debt, but it still makes it very stressful and uncomfortable for the family to be receiving the constant bills and dealing with collectors at the hospital, while mourning of the recent death of their loved one. Because of this concern, many lower income patients fear going into a hospital in the first place when they are very ill, and instead choose to die at home, either in formal hospice care provided by community health agencies or religious organizations, or just being cared for by close family or friends.

Major Decisions that Must Be Made at the End of Life
The care given to a patient at the end of their life is called palliative care. The National Institute on Aging defines palliative care as "the specialized medical care for people living with a serious illness, such as cancer or heart failure. Patients in palliative care may receive medical care for their symptoms, or palliative care, along with treatment intended to cure their serious illness. Palliative care is meant to enhance a person's current care by focusing on quality of life for them and their family." There are physicians who specialize in palliative care
and many of them belong to the American Academy of Hospice and Palliative Care. There are three major issues of medical ethics that the AHPC has defined that become relevant in making the medical decisions for a patient at the end of their life. These three issues are explained below and the position statements of the AHPC are presented.

Artificial Nutrition and Hydration Near the End of Life

This is when the patient is administered nutrition and water intravenously. "Artificial nutrition and hydration (ANH) were originally developed to provide short-term support for patients who were acutely ill., and the consensus is that for patients near the end of life, ANH is unlikely to prolong life and can potentially lead to medical complications and increase suffering."

Palliative Sedation

This is when doctors put an end of life patient into an induced coma. "Palliative care supports patients whose diseases are associated with significant burden. Distressing symptoms exist on a spectrum from the most easily treated to the most refractory. Although preservation of awareness at the end of life is viewed as a priority for many, for some, the relief of symptoms may outweigh the desire to be conscious."

Withholding and Withdrawing Nonbeneficial Medical Interventions

"Palliative care seeks to relieve suffering associated with life-limiting illness. As illness progresses, there also may be times when the burdens of medical interventions outweigh their benefits, when the intervention is nonbeneficial, or when its use is inconsistent with the patient's goals." At that point, doctors will typically approach the family to discuss withholding certain treatments or withdrawing interventions that have been started. The concept of "pulling the plug" falls into the category of withdrawing nonbeneficial medical interventions. This is a major decision for a surrogate decision maker to make, and very often conflicts with the principles of major religions. Indeed, many cases have gone to court when one member of the family wants to continue treatment, even if the patient remains in a coma, and other members of the family want to either withhold treatment or withdraw treatment. This is why the Advanced Directive is so important because it clarifies the patient's wishes at the time of death as to what interventions should be followed.

Meeting the Expectations of Patients: The Perspective of a Palliative Care Nurse

Certainly, one of the most important healthcare providers attending to the end of life patient is the nurse. These nurses are trained in intensive care nursing, and they are monitoring the health status of the patient from minute to minute. In a recent workshop presented to palliative care nurses at the Physicians' Education Resource's 3rd Annual School of Nursing Oncology meeting in 2019, Brianna Kirkland, RN, a member of the clinical staff of Sangre de Cristo Hospice and Palliative Care, discussed these important guidelines of how to meet the expectations of patients and their families.

She stated that "before discussing a patient's prognosis, nurses must ensure they make no assumptions when it comes to the patient's or the patient's family's understanding of the state of their disease." Often, patients and their family members are not fully aware of the full diagnosis and prognosis of the patient. Often, the patient or a family member needs to ask the doctor to be upfront with full disclosure of what the doctor knows.

"The second step, Nurse Kirkland continues, is for nurses to respect patient autonomy, support decision-making, and provide personalized care. To do this, Kirkland says, healthcare staff should ensure that an advanced care plan (ACP) is discussed and documented; share information across settings and teams throughout their e-health records; and minimize fragmentation of care by supporting one doctor or health professional to coordinate care of the terminally or chronically ill patients."

"The third step is to ensure medical treatment decisions are reflective and respect the patient's best interest. Knowing when to withhold or limit treatment that is inappropriate or potentially harmful to the patient is a key component of exceptional end-of-life care," she stated.

"In the fourth step, nurses must ensure that proper management of symptoms is an ongoing component of end-of-life care. Of note, symptoms can change as the patient's condition may progress, and new or ongoing treatments may also contribute to this."

Lastly, Kirkland recommended for the healthcare staff to support the patient's family, their culture and their religious beliefs. "Providing support to family members and significant others before and after death is an essential part of providing good end-of-life care."

"Their involvement — with patient consent – in discussions around the prognosis, the goals of care, and the Advanced Care Plan are all important to this support," she added. "It becomes essential if the patient lacks the capacity to make their own preferences known."

The Decision to Move the Patient to Hospice and the Reasonable Expectations

Very often, the doctors caring for a patient in the hospital, either with the consent of the patient or the consent of the family, decide that the patient should be transitioned to hospice care. Hospice care is defined by the National Institute on Aging, a major agency that supports the elderly, as "both a service and a philosophy. Hospice embraces that quality of life is much more important than quantity and emphasizes caring rather than curing. The primary goal of hospice care is to provide comprehensive care to the terminally ill and their families, helping them to continue life as normally as possible." Hospice care generally is provided in the patient's home or the home of a loved one or friend, but some patients choose to a hospice facility, where the same personal care is provided round the clock by experienced nurses and doctors. The most common type of hospice for the end of life patient is continuous care home hospice, where a hospice nurse remains with the patient at their bedside to monitor the medical equipment that has been sent home with the patient and also monitor the status of the patient. Often, the nurse is supported by a palliative care physician who will visit the patient in their home and confer with the nurse to make sure that everything is being done to ensure that the patient is as comfortable as they can be.

According to Emily Davis, Hospice Marketing Manager for Bayada Home Health Care, the goal of hospice is "to maintain the quality of life for the patient while addressing their pain and symptoms, while also providing emotional support to the patient and their family. Hospice is provided in a team approach to make sure that the medical needs of the patient are met and that the patient remains comforted and serene."

And maintaining a peaceful and serene environment is the greatest expectation that a patient and their family has for hospice care. In addition, the patient and family expect dedicated care by the hospice team including empathy, support, understanding, and encouragement. In addition, the family expects guidance with what will need to be done after the death occurs, and how to find bereavement support. It is very common for the hospice nurse to call the funeral home to arrange for the deceased person to be moved from their home to the funeral home, as well as helping the family to contact the medical equipment company to remove the equipment that was used in the home during the hospice care.

And so, it is clear that patients and their families have reasonable expectations throughout the lifetime of the patient, and as situations change throughout the lifecycle, those expectations change as well.

In the next and final section of the book, we will turn our attention to the role of the patient/provider relationship, the role of a changing healthcare delivery system, and finally, if patient centered care is indeed being provided to all patients in this country.

PART FIVE
STRENGTHS AND THREATS

Chapter Nineteen

The Impact of Communication
By De'Andre Alexander, Airiana Michelle Davis, Anat Ferleger, and Juhi Patel

This chapter will focus on the impact of the provider/patient relationship and how it impacts patient-centered care in the mind of the patient. The chapter will explore how trust and honest communication between patients and providers is essential in fostering a positive patient-centered care experience.

Patient-Provider Relationship
Central to practicing medicine, the patient-provider relationship encompasses their shared decision-making as a result of the provider serving a patient's medical needs. In the United States, there has been a recent change in the ideal model for a healthcare provider and patient relationship. Before healthcare systems used paternalistic models, the providers made decisions for a patient without consent. The provider believed their decisions had the patient's best intentions. However, most would argue that paternalism will allow providers to withhold valuable information with the assumption of knowing the patient's desires while making decisions. Thus, other models have replaced paternalistic models with an emphasis on respect for patients' freedom and shared decision-making. A positive patient-provider relationship is best accomplished by open communication, a sense of empathy, and a cooperative attitude from both parties.

Importance of Patient-Provider Relationship

Since the early 1900s, studies have analyzed a patient-provider relationship as essential in healthcare. The standard patient-provider relationship in the United States may include a 10–15-minute appointment with very little detailed information. Most patients come in and out of the doctor's office unsatisfied and defeated. They want to negotiate the healthcare system effectively while being treated with respect. Patients desire to trust the competence and efficacy of their caregivers. When the patient is satisfied with their care, they will better adhere to treatment from the providers. So, the patient-provider relationship can impact the treatment's success. Therefore, an effective patient-provider relationship can improve patient satisfaction, health outcomes, medical care, and the overall patient experience.

Correlation to Patient-Centered Care

The majority of patients prefer a patient-centered type of care within facilities. The strength of the patient-provider relationship directly impacts the kind of care offered. When providing patient-centered care, the patient-provider relationship is strong, defined by a high level of patient satisfaction. Thus, providers must be flexible in addressing variations in patient preferences. Because patient satisfaction is exceptionally high irrespective, it can be challenging to measure their overall expectations. So, providers should better understand how their patient's expectations and satisfaction relate by communicating and building a relationship. It means there is an ongoing dialogue between the provider and their patient; they have set expectations and communication preferences and have worked towards strengthening their patient-provider relationship.

Communication Between Patient and Provider Is Essential

Productive and proper communication between patients and providers is an essential element of healthcare which, in some cases, can make a difference between life and death. Providers who facilitate open communication can develop rapport with their patients, obtain a complete history, and enhance the prospect of more accurate diagnoses. In return, this can help improve treatment plans that benefit the patient's long-term health, improving patient outcomes. Effective communication is the foundation of healthcare. When done correctly, it leads to greater patient satisfaction, patient compliance, and the ability for patients, family, and care teams to work effectively together. It begins with healthcare organizations taking a step back and recognizing that listening is the only way to communicate effectively with patients. Physicians have incredible knowledge unused when they rush from appointment to appointment without proper communication tactics. It is a physician's job to put patients at ease and make them feel heard and safe enough to disclose issues they are facing. Patient satisfaction will not execute when a physician is being rushed and not prioritizing their relationships with patients.

Barriers in Communication

A lack of trust is one of the most significant barriers to communication between patients and providers. Many patients do not feel comfortable with their physicians and withhold disclosing sensitive information. Some reasons a patient may withhold medical details are as follows:

- A patient may feel intimidated by their provider
- They feel as though they won't be listened to
- They feel disrespected
- They have physical and psychological trauma
- They question medical advice in general

Language is another common barrier. While healthcare institutions are required to provide interpreters, they often fall short or are not culturally competent. Providers are also often pushed over their limits. Systems force providers to see far more patients in a shift than they have time to see. It can lead to a lack of effective communication. Providers cannot establish rapport or provide crucial health information, which diminishes the patient quality of care.

Strategies for Improving Healthcare Communication
There are a variety of actions providers can take to help improve their communication with patients during a patient encounter. Recommendations include following an established model to help providers effectively communicate with patients and cover all of their bases. A few of the recommended models are as follows.

AIDET is a tactic used around the country. The Studer Group developed AIDET, which includes five fundamental principles of patient communication. They are as follows: providers must first *acknowledge* their patients, positively greet them, be attentive throughout the visit, and *introduce* themselves to the patient. Also, they should have a reasonable expectation of the *duration* of the stay. By the end of the visit, providers should give patients a proper *explanation*, information, and understanding of the discussion. Lastly, the provider should end the examination with a "*Thank you.*" The provider should show appreciation to the patient for their cooperation and communication.

The "BATHE" technique is another recommended technique for physicians as it helps ensure that providers have covered all their bases. This tactic includes discussing a patient's *background* (general information about their life), *affect* (how their emotions affect their overall health issue), *troubling* (what is it about their situation that is the most overwhelming/frightening), *handling* (how they are processing their condition) and *empathy* (reflect what you hear).

The RESPECT model is another model generally used to help physicians become more aware of their own biases and to help them build a rapport with patients from a whole host of different backgrounds. This model includes seven aspects; connection, empathy, support, partnership, explanations, cultural competence, and trust.

While these tactics play an essential role in effective patient-provider interaction, there are some other actions providers can take to help further improve their relationships and communication with patients. Staying seated throughout office visits can help to build trust with patients. It creates the illusion of a more intimate visit and allows patients to feel as though they are on the same level as the provider, which can help ease the patient's anxiety.

Open-ended questions are another tactic that physicians may use. It allows for a more empathetic conversation and helps to build rapport. Providers can also make it a point to speak a plain language to their patients. They should explain to patients medical terminology in a way the patient can understand to help ease one's anxiety. Healthcare facilities should also prioritize hiring culturally competent staff and interpreters available. It helps to ensure that all patients receive culturally competent and effective healthcare. Ensuring communication is confidential is also an essential aspect of improving healthcare communication. When patients feel that the patient care team will not keep the information shared, they are far less likely to share issues they face.

All of these more minor tactics, as well as the models discussed, can help ensure equal and effective communication between providers and patients. While these models can be overwhelming, it is critical to remember four essential components of practical and caring communication skills which should be in mind throughout every visit; comfort, acceptance, responsiveness, and empathy.

Providers Communicating with Low Health Literacy Patients

Health literacy is the degree to which individuals can locate, process, and understand basic information and resources needed to make appropriate health-related decisions for themselves. Health literacy helps people discover quality health care and services and maintain their wellness. However, health providers often overestimate their patient's level of health literacy. According to a resource provider OneOp, low health literacy is common among older adults, minorities, people with language barriers, and low socioeconomic populations. Patients with low health literacy may struggle with applying for health insurance coverage, sharing medical history, filling out the information, understanding medication directions, and managing their health issues. So, health professionals should be aware of their patient's health literacy to communicate information best. Providers can practice listening intently, asking open-ended questions, and encouraging patients to share viable information. They can increase the use of simple terminology and limit medical jargon use. And providers can organize essential information, provide printed-out materials, and slowly present five or fewer pieces of data to ensure the patient will understand.

Overall, providers and professionals can best communicate health concerns by connecting with their patient's backgrounds, becoming their advocates, and preparing to promote understanding between the patient and provider.

Patient-Provider Relationships Improve Healthcare Facilities

It is no surprise that fostering a friendly patient-provider relationship can improve the patient's experience and the facility's credibility and promote loyalty to the specific practice. There are four steps healthcare leaders can practice during patient interactions to establish trust. The first step is simply to practice active listening. It is sometimes easy for physicians who meet with many patients daily to overlook the small details of what the patient is saying and only listen enough to fill out their medical charts. Active listening helps prevent this from happening because it requires your undivided attention to the patient and listening to the words they are saying and the tone, body language, and emotions. By doing this, patients will feel not only valued but heard as well. The second step is creating a connection with the patient. The physician needs to hear more than just the science and symptoms. For example, physicians must listen to the health concerns and goals of the patient and consider external factors contributing to their health concerns. The third step is giving and acknowledging nonverbal communication. Words are important, but things like your posture, level of eye contact, and even reactions are signifying factors to prove or disprove that you genuinely care about the patient. When these actions align with the physician's words, they improve the patient's trust. The last step is relaying the understanding of patient concerns and goals by the provider to the patient. After the physician has actively listened to the patient, established a personal connection, and showed empathetic and intentional body language, a tangible way to conclude the conversation is by repeating the patient's concerns and goals aloud. Doing this will indicate that the physician has been paying attention and understands the patient's reasoning.

Conclusion
In short, the definition of a patient-care provider relationship is when there is open communication, empathy, and a cooperative attitude between both parties. This dynamic is extremely important in the healthcare industry because of how fast clinical appointments have become with very little

information sometimes being exchanged. A healthy patient-care provider relationship will make the patient more comfortable to open up about pressing issues, increasing patient satisfaction, experience, and even medical care provided. Patient-centered care is also vital when the patient/provider relationship is strong. In other words, the patient/provider relationship directly impacts the care provided. The more comfortable the patient feels during the clinical appointment will ultimately allow the physician to thoroughly analyze the patient's concerns and create a more tailored plan of action to help the patient.

Chapter Twenty

The Impact of Corporate Medicine
By Courtney Pokallus and Bob Kieserman

In 1990, there were 6,650 hospitals in the United States. In 2016, there were 5,530. That is because around 2010, a new chapter in healthcare management began to take place. Between 2010 and 2017, the country saw the growth of hospital systems with major hospitals in various regions of the country buying smaller hospitals and/or merging with similar size hospitals to form large regional healthcare systems. And as part of the game plan of the hospital systems to become the major supplier of healthcare, doctors in private practice were approached to sell their practices to the healthcare systems. At first, many doctors, especially older very established private practitioners, resisted, but the offers by the hospital systems were so lucrative, that the doctors accepted the offers. Some of the older doctors retired at that point, while others who wanted to continue to practice medicine became employees for the first time in their medical careers. For those doctors, life became very different. No longer were the doctors making decisions about the business operations of their practices. That now became the responsibility of the hospital systems who took over. The doctors were employees and their job was just to practice medicine. The hospital systems took care of everything else.

At the same time, the hospital systems placed many protocols on the doctors and their staffs. Important protocols like how much time a doctor should spend with a patient, how many patients the staff needs to schedule in a certain day, whether a patient should see a doctor or a physician assistant or a certified nurse practitioner, and many other rules that became the universal protocols of all system-owned offices. At the same time that the not for profit hospital systems were growing, for-profit healthcare corporations who owned hospitals and created their own network of employed doctors were quietly increasing in number. Over the past two years, the hospital systems and these for-profit corporations have continued to grow even larger. This has been called the rise of corporate medicine. The big question is whether this change has benefited the patient or whether it has not.

The Presence of Healthcare Corporations
A recent study by the Physician Advocacy Institute and Avalere Health, a consulting firm, found that the pandemic actually accelerated this trend of corporate medicine companies acquiring physician practices with over 25,000 physicians leaving their private practices and joining these hospitals and companies since the pandemic began. It is estimated that in the beginning of 2021, nearly 70% of physicians were employed with just 3 out of 10 doctors still practicing independently.

The Doctors Are Not Happy
Late last year, the Physicians Advocacy Institute sent an open letter to members of Congress to warn against this "major shift toward the corporatization of healthcare". According to the open letter, if Congress did not take action to monitor the activities of these big hospital systems and prevent them from reducing the clinical autonomy of doctors to provide high-quality, cost effective care for patients, this could have major implications for the overall American healthcare system and definitely affect the welfare of patients across the country.

This is the real issue. With the change of how healthcare is delivered, under the model of corporate medicine, doctors have lost the ability to practice medicine as they were trained to do and to make clinical decisions for the good of the patient, and not for the good of the bottom line of the companies that now own their offices.

An article titled *Financial Profit in Medicine: A Position Paper From the American College of Physicians* brings up multiple points about corporate medicine and its effects on patient-centered care and the patient/physician relationship.

The article relates that "in 2013, neurosurgeon Russell J. Andrews blamed the nation's health care crisis on two factors: the erosion of the patient–physician relationship, in which physicians take personal responsibility to ensure that patients receive the best possible care, and the transition from medicine as a humanitarian function of society to a revenue stream for healthcare professionals, drug and medical device companies, hospitals, and insurance companies"

We believe that these two factors go hand in hand. From the way the healthcare system in the United States has evolved, it seems that the only way we have arrived at this revenue centered system is by deteriorating the patient-physician relationship. There is no other way to make the amount of money that hospital systems are making other than compromising on the way physicians are able to take care of patients. To many patients, it seems like physicians are always running around, overbooked and only able to give each patient a few minutes of their time. A doctor cannot possibly resolve a patient's concerns correctly when the doctor is only allotted a small amount of time with each patient. Physicians are taking on many patients at one time mostly for the reason that more patients at a time means more money coming into the office. This system has destroyed the patient-physician relationship in the name of generating more money.

The paper also states that "the American health care system of the 21st century resembles the medical-industrial complex that drew Arnold Relman's concern in the 1980s. What many imagine to be a lean, market-based system is actually bloated, complex, and fragmented, increasingly directed toward generating profit. The same profit motive that can encourage new thinking and innovation can also cultivate the profit-over-patients orientation warned of in medicine's historic oaths and professional guidelines. Ultimately, professionalism, medical ethics, and the patient–physician relationship must guide how physicians navigate the business side of medicine. Nonprofits must act like nonprofits and have a community-oriented mission. Likewise the private equity firms and investor-owned healthcre organizations must focus on the needs of patients and not just shareholders. Most importantly, physicians should not have a financial stake in an organization with which they have a referral relationship."

When you think about it, the amount of money being made could be used to further expand our healthcare system, creating new devices, new treatments that can further help the patient. It is true that we have scientists who are innovating new ways of healthcare, but the large hospital systems are not the ones doing the innovating. There are some hospitals that are renovating and changing the ways hospitals are supposed to look, from gloomy and cold to looking like a spa, but unfortunately there are not many hospitals doing that. Most keep the uncomfortable chairs, vinyl flooring and white walls, not expanding and innovating new ways to do healthcare. They are only overbooking physicians, causing them to burnout, leading to a strained relationship between patient and physician, all for the purpose of funding corporate greed.

Hospital systems need to be putting their efforts into improving the way healthcare is provided in their facilities. In order to reach a system of better quality healthcare, there needs to be an implementation of innovative and new techniques to enhance the patient and physician experience. We need to move away from the current system that we have in place, overworking physicians and underwhelming patients, in order to change the way that patients are given healthcare and overall enhance the healthcare system.

How This Affects Patients
And so, we see that the big hospital systems and the for-profit healthcare companies, because they are seeking high financial returns in reimbursements and fees for service, have

pressured their employed doctors to see patients more often for followup visits, order more tests that the third party insurance companies will pay for, and a push for virtual visits rather than live in-office visits, since they can charge the same for a virtual visit as they do for an in-office visit, but the virtual visit usually ends up being shorter and easier for the doctor. In addition, practices are being told to schedule more appointments with the physician assistant or the certified nurse practitioner instead of with the doctor, but charge the same for the visit.

The increase in physicians being employed by hospitals has proportionately compromised the patient-physician relationship. This shift has caused a huge change as patients are not the top priority anymore, making money is. Many of the hospital systems that took over the small practices are investor owned. These for-profit hospitals also tend to be more expensive and charge at higher rates than Medicare, but have a larger proportion of uninsured patients compared to non-for-profit healthcare centers. This means they predominantly care about making as much money as possible, not the care of the patients. The change has caused patients to get less time with doctors, less quality of care and an overall higher costing service. The patient-physician relationship is vital to having a good patient-centered care system, but this relationship and patient-centered practice has been damaged since the influx of hospital systems. Patient-centered care focuses on both a healthy practice for the patient and for the physician. This includes improving access to care, preventing burn out for the physician, integrating family and patient into healthcare decisions and overall improving the visit for both patient and physician. This corporate medicine approach has not only added cost to healthcare, but deteriorated the patient-centered ideals that are crucial to a seamless experience for everyone involved.

Patients have also complained that doctors spend more time looking at the computer during a visit, than talking to the patient and examining them. This is due to new protocols connected with the use of electronic medical records. Because many offices are scheduling three patients or more for the same appointment time, the doctor is rushed and in some cases, no longer fully examining a patient, as they once did. We have come to learn and appreciate that the doctors are not happy with the situation. They are doing the best they can, but they know they are not giving their patients the same personal attention they once did. In some cases, this new way of practicing medicine has caused physician burnout with many excellent doctors retiring earlier than planned or leaving medicine altogether and getting into a different career path. For many older patients, in particular, the doctors who have cared for them for decades, are deciding they have had enough, and are retiring, leaving the older patients to find new doctors and start new relationships late in life, when they need doctors the most.

What Can Patients Do?
There are really two major things patients can do to help the situation. The first is to be understanding and verbally support your doctors. Tell them how much you appreciate them, tell them that you understand they are under new pressures that they never had before, and try to be less demanding on what you know should be, but just can't be right now. The other thing that patients can do is to let the hospital systems and/or the healthcare companies know that you value your doctors and that they need to give as much autonomy to the doctors as they need to practice medicine the way the doctors want for the benefit of their patients. Patients can make a difference. The large systems and corporations are big on surveys. They send them out all of the time, especially after an office or virtual visit. Be sure to be honest about your experiences and let them know that doctors, even though they are now employees, need to be able to practice medicine with full decision making powers, deciding what is best for the patient including what tests need to be ordered, what specialists they need to see, how often they need to return for followup visits, and how necessary it is for certain medications to be prescribed or not prescribed.

Corporate medicine has changed the way healthcare is delivered. As healthcare has shifted to more of a business structure than patient centered, it is taking time away from patients just to squeeze in more patients to make more money. In order to make it a more efficient system for both patients and staff, we need to restore the patient-physician relationship and ensure that all parties, both the providers and the patients, are content in the way treatment is delivered.

Chapter Twenty One

Is Patient Centered Care Being Practiced?
By Bob Kieserman

In 2004, as part of class of an introductory course I was teaching in The Principles of Healthcare Administration at Arcadia University's School of Global Business, where I served as Chair of the Healthcare Administration Department for over 20 years, I created a poster that many years later became the basis for The Power of the Patient Project, the organization that I began along with some of my students and now has become a multi-level digital portal for healthcare information.

This poster speaks to healthcare providers letting them know through a patient's voice what patients expect from their providers. It is based on the Patient Bill of Rights, a fascinating and well conceived document which was drafted and adopted in 1973 by the American Hospital Association. According to the AHA, The Patient Bill of Rights "was developed with the expectation that hospitals and health care institutions would support these rights in the interest of delivering effective patient care." In its announcement of the document, the AHA encouraged facilities and medical offices to translate and/or simplify the bill of rights to meet the needs of their specific patient populations and to make patient rights and responsibilities understandable to patients and their families. The AHA also reminded facilities that "a patient's rights can be exercised on the patient's behalf by a designated surrogate or proxy decision-maker if the patient lacks decision-making capacity, is legally incompetent, or is a minor."

As we conclude this book, I want to share this poster with you, and then make some final points to answer the ultimate question of whether patient centered care is really being practiced in America.

Read this carefully, and see how well you relate to what it says.

I Am a Patient ….

and I want to be treated with respect by your practice.

I want you to talk to me in a way that I can understand everything you are saying to me. Please ask me if I really understand what you are telling me, and I will confirm for you whether I do or not. Please do not be offended if I want to tape record what you say to me or bring someone with me to be my "second set of ears". This is only so that I can make sure I hear everything you need to explain to me.

Please have compassion for the fact that I am scared, often not knowing if something is seriously wrong with me when I come to see you, and please be sensitive to this fear of mine.

Please have patience for my questions when I ask them and really listen to what I am asking you.

When I arrive for an appointment, I would appreciate not having to wait more than 15 minutes in your waiting room before I am taken into an examination room. While I am waiting, it would be nice if there were current magazines to read and maybe a television to watch to ease the anxiety.

Once I am in the examination room, I would appreciate being seen within 20 minutes. I certainly understand that sometimes you fall behind with your schedule because each patient has different demands for your time. However, could you please have someone from your office come into the examination room periodically and let me know what is going on in terms of your schedule, so that I can be more understanding about the delay, rather than becoming more and more impatient waiting for you?

I need you to know that sitting alone in the examination room can be a real frightening experience especially if you have instruments in sight that can start to make my mind worry. Perhaps, you can try to make the examination room as pleasant as possible while I wait for you. After all, if it is necessary for me to wait for you, I would like to be pleasantly entertained while I wait.

I expect you to be respectful of my privacy. I become very upset when I am sitting in the waiting room or even in examination room and I can hear everything that you or the receptionist or nurse is saying in the next room or over the phone to other patients, hospitals, or physicians. I am upset because I know that if I am hearing this about others, others who are sitting in the waiting room or the next examination rooms are probably hearing something confidential about me.

Therefore, I think it's fair for me to expect you to provide some type of system where confidential patient information cannot be heard by other patients.

Please be honest with me about my medical condition and the possibility of pain as you examine me.

There are many times that I really need to speak with you. Please try to call me back within a reasonable time when I call you, day or night. Whenever I have undergone tests or procedures, please also have you or someone from your office call me back to discuss the results, and not just send me a letter in the mail.

Please hire competent, compassionate people to support your practice, who will be sympathetic to my need to see you or speak with you, and who will work with me in terms of insurance claims and referrals that I need.

Overall, I would like to feel like a guest of your practice, and be treated by you and your staff as if your practice depends upon me, because it does.

To me, this is the essence of patient centered care, and all of these patient rights have been mentioned and explained throughout the book. The themes of speaking in a language that the patient understands including not using jargon that can confuse the patient or family members; having empathy and compassion for the patient's anxiety, especially when the patient may not know what the diagnosis will be and how it will be treated; making the patient feel that they are being listened to and believed during the visit; showing courtesy and respect for the patient's time, and not making them wait longer than necessary to be seen; paying attention to confidentiality and respecting a patient's right of privacy to what is said to the provider and what is shared with others; being proactive about a patient's right to full disclosure of their medical condition and the risks of a treatment; being respectful that when a patient needs to reach a provider, that the provider responds by phone or through a patient portal; paying attention to who sits at the front desk as support staff and making sure that those support and clinical members of your practice are kind, considerate, and helpful; and always staying conscious of the fact that patients matter and whatever your hospital or practice can do to serve the patient is what everyone involved in patient care must do.

This is patient centered care.

The Ultimate Question
And so, we get to the end of our book and answer the question of whether patient centered care is truly being practiced by providers, administrators, support staff, and others connected with our healthcare. I believe it is. I believe that with the pressures that have been placed on our doctors, nurses, therapists, physician assistants, and others on the healthcare team, they are doing the best job they can. Everyone working in healthcare today is a true hero.

However, I do remain concerned with the influence of corporate medicine on patient centered care. I am concerned about things like the pressures placed on providers such as only having a limited amount of time with a patient, keeping medical records that must be entered during the visit taking away eye to eye contact with the patient, coping with constraints placed on providers by insurance companies, and the challenges of providing quality care to all members of our society, regardless of their economic background, education, age, gender, or where they live. I am concerned with whether these issues will ever be fully addressed, or whether the patient/provider relationship will become even more strained. I hope not. I hope that the next generation of providers and administrators will make sure that patients always come first, and that patient centered care will always remain the major mission of everyone practicing medicine. One of the best ways to guarantee this is for patients to understand that they have rights, that they have a voice, and that they have an obligation to work with their providers and to respect their providers, and to help everyone in healthcare to do their job with dedication and with respect for all patients.

About the Authors

De'Andre Alexander is a senior at Marquette University on the premed track double majoring in Biological Sciences and Psychology. He also currently works as a medical scribe at Cancer Treatment of America where he has built an authentic and personal bond with not only the physicians, but also the patients as well. He aspires to attend medical school and become a neurosurgeon. De'Andre regards Dr. Ben Carson, the noted neurosurgeon and author as one of his major role models.

Riham Alwaely is from Kansas City, and is currently a junior at the University of Missouri-Kansas City pursuing a Bachelors degree in Chemistry and a double minor in Biology and Business Administration. She plans to become a dentist and aspires to bring about confident smiles in people through oral medicine. She is an advocate for patients and has a great interest in the sociology of medicine.

Hugo Amador is an undergraduate student at Cornell University. He is currently studying cellular & molecular biology, journalism, and Latin American studies. After being born and raised in Honduras, Hugo moved to the United States in flee against gang violence where he has worked with many organizations in research/advocacy – primarily towards immigrant and refugee populations. He has given many TEDx talks, having his talks published with global organizations, and has also worked on clinical research within immigrant populations in the New York metropolitan area along with an infectious disease team. Hugo is the recipient of prestigious and competitive academic fellowships, such as the Cornell Commitment Fellowship, and is the founder of Hugo's Movement, a not-for-profit that advocates for the access to equitable healthcare, education, and liberty of victims of war and gang violence, primarily immigrant children and adolescents.

Aaliya Anaya is a graduate of California State University, Channel Islands with a Bachelor's degree in Health Science. During her undergraduate program, she was an intern with the California Department of Public Health where she was inspired to be in the field of public health. Her goal is to pursue practical frameworks to build a foundation of evidence through research and to promote that evidence through advocacy in order to improve population health. She has a passion for addressing the systemic social issues affecting underserved communities through policy change. She is planning to pursue a Master's in Public Health with a focus in Health Policy and Management.

Abigail Arient is a recent graduate of Stetson University with a Bachelor of Science in Health Science and a Bachelor of Art in History. With interests in health promotion, patient advocacy, and accessibility she hopes to pursue a career in physical or occupational therapy. She is also a Certified Pharmacy Technician and a medical billing coordinator and has received numerous academic honors.

Olivia Arkell is a recent graduate from Hamline University who studied psychology, philosophy, neuroscience, and political science. She has a strong interest in biomedical ethics and the psychotherapeutic value of psychedelics. Olivia is always looking for ways she can expand her understanding on how we can transform the way we treat mental illness in the clinical setting. She demonstrates this passion through researching and interpreting literature then translating it into a short article/blog form that is easy, reliable, and comprehensible for the general public to read.

Emelia Behnan is currently pursuing a Master of Public Health degree at the University of Southern California, with a focus on community health promotion. Emelia has a background in healthcare in the areas of health information management and patient billing. She has also volunteered her talents and time to several organizations to help community members with English proficiency and navigating the healthcare delivery system.

Dima Bischoff-Hashem is an undergraduate at Rutgers University pursuing a double major in public health and computer science. She interned with The Power of the Patient last summer, and she is particularly interested in healthcare policy and affordability in healthcare. Last semester, she worked in a lab in her school's department of cell biology and neuroscience, researching treatments for traumatic brain injuries. She also interned with three social work professors at Rutgers to contribute research for their publication on environmental justice. Dima hopes to take classes in addiction policy and public health law and aims to affect policy change in her career. Dima is also a contributor to *Today's Patient*, our online magazine.

Julianna Celestin is an ambitious-driven graduate from Florida State University, where she has obtained degrees in Family & Child Sciences and Public Health with a Minor in Child Development. She is currently pursuing a Master of Health Services Administration in Healthcare and later a Juris Master with a specific concentration in Healthcare. Her aspiration is to become a Healthcare Administrator and Researcher focused on strengthening systems solutions to public health, comprehensive health systems, and health care problems. Julianna's focus is improving access to healthcare. She is passionately committed to progressively improving the social efficiency and quality of healthcare services that are being provided and not provided to those in the underserved, underrepresented, and vulnerable populations.

Airiana Michelle Davis is a graduate of Georgia State University with a Bachelor of Science degree in Public Health and a minor in Chemistry. During her time at GSU, Airiana was not only committed to her academics but she was involved within the community, serving on the Executive Board in one of her eight organizations. She has the heart to minister and the experience working with various non-profit organizations, like Books for Africa and the Second Harvest of South Georgia Food Bank. Airiana also has a background with years of experience in the arts as a model, dancer, artist, designer, instrumentalist, and creative director. With her background in art and knowledge as a public health graduate, Airiana desires to bridge the gap between both to serve, seek intervention, and improve the lifestyles of individuals in underrepresented minority communities. One of Airiana's goals is to collaborate with national leaders to develop, implement, and administer creative art services in public health systems for equality, health promotion, behavior change, and mental health on a global scale.

Anat Ferleger is a recent graduate from American University with a Bachelor's degree in Psychology and Public Health, on the pre-med track. Throughout college she spent her time volunteering at a local fire station as an Emergency Medical Technician, as well as working with SOUL programs running workshops focused on academic, athletic and professional enrichment opportunities for low income DC youth. During the Covid-19 crisis, she volunteered administering vaccines at clinics around Washington, D.C. In her free time, she enjoys traveling and hiking with her Goldendoodle, Chloe. In the next year, Anat is planning to apply to medical school and hopes to use her interest in medical sociology to better herself as a physician.

Bansi H. Kakadiya has a bachelor's degree in Biology from the University of Georgia and is currently pursuing a Master's degree in Biomedical Sciences. Through her education, she wants to help people in need in the rural parts of the country. She enjoys volunteering for food banks, hospitals, and homeless shelters in Georgia in her leisure time. She is currently working to open a nonprofit organization in India to provide education for girls.

Bansari Kheni is pursuing a Master's of Public Health with a concentration in Population Health at Wright State University. Bansari is a dentist by background and has experience of more than three years of treating patients. She became interested in studying public health during her junior year of undergraduate school as she is someone who has always prioritized health and serving the community. Her current goal is to give better health outcomes to the community. She would like to see the potential impact of her work by giving some unique concepts on public health in the community by improving the health of individuals and society.

Robert H. Kieserman is the Founding Executive Director of The Power of the Patient Project. Bob served as the Program Director of the Health Administration Program and was a member of the senior faculty at the Arcadia University School of Global Business for over 20 years. Throughout his 35 year career, Bob taught and mentored thousands of men and women preparing them for careers as physicians, nurses, rehab therapists, hospital administrators, nursing home administrators, and medical practice administrators. He earned his MBA from the Fox School of Business at Temple University and his MLIS from the Rutgers University School of Communication and Information. Prior to joining Arcadia, Bob was the CEO of one of the country's leading continuing medical education companies for over 15 years, and prior to that served as Assistant to the Deans of the Temple University School of Medicine. He is the author of four books on medical practice management and over 200 articles on the issues of healthcare management and patient rights. Bob's passion is educating patients about their rights and empowering patients to be better consumers of the healthcare delivery system.

Mason La Fleur is a senior at Grand Valley State University preparing for a career in healthcare administration and studying Health Communications. He serves as the President of the GVSU Health Communication Club, is a member of GVSU Students for Choice, and the GVSU Beekeeping club. Upon graduation, he plans to pursue a Master's in Health Administration with the career goal of working in a healthcare facility. In his free time, Mason enjoys reading, working out, spending time with friends, and watching movies.

Yu-Tung Lu also goes by Anna. She is currently in professional year 1 in the Doctor of Pharmacy program at Massachusetts College of Pharmacy. Her future goal is to do the residency program after graduating and put emphasis on patient-centered care. She believes that asides from the medications that pharmacists place importance on, that other factors such as social environment, mental health, and others significantly impact a patient's health.

Juhi Patel is a third-year student at the University of South Carolina Honors College as part of the BARSC-MD program, an accelerated 7-year M.D. track, with concentrations in Cellular Biology and Neuroscience. She has aspirations to become a physician scientist and work toward more holistic healthcare. She is interested in health advocacy and patient-centered care, with experience in both clinical care and health policy.

Courtney Pokallus is a Healthcare Administration Major with a minor in Global Public Health at Arcadia University. She has also completed two seasons competitively swimming for Arcadia and has experience volunteering for multiple organizations including the One Project and her local public library. With a great interest in the healthcare system in the United States, Courtney is committed to advocating for patients rights. As the Associate Director of Provider Outreach and Education for The Power of the Patient Project, Courtney also serves as the Project Coordinator for MedFocus Research & Publishing.

Michelle Powell is an undergraduate student at Michigan State University majoring in Human Biology with plans to become a physician or PA. She is passionate about writing stories to help people that led her to join her school's Her Campus chapter. With her desire for journalism, Michelle is a member of the editorial staff of *Today's Patient*. Her focus is to explain medicine and medical issues to help patients with any misunderstandings they may have about the healthcare system.

Regina Rush is a Research Analyst, who studies state, local, and educational technology solution trends throughout the United States. She received her Bachelor of Science degree in Sociology with a minor in Anthropology from the Florida A&M University. For the past year and a half, Rush has spent her time doing market research. Regina plans to obtain her doctoral degree in Sociology.

Anooshka Shukla has a Bachelors of Science and with a major in Public Health from Massachusetts College of Pharmacy and Health Sciences (MCPHS) and is currently pursuing Masters of Public Health from the same university, with plans to graduate this summer. She worked as a Teaching Fellow for Citizen School in Boston, MA which works to help inner city students achieve their full potential. She assisted senior citizens in an adult day care center providing health care information. Anooshka also volunteered in a local pharmacy assisting with logistics and customer service. Being passionate about public health, Anooshka is always excited to empower patients, especially in mental health area.

Tasfia Wahid is a graduate of Stony Brook University with a Bachelors degree in Sociology and a minor in Biology and Chemistry, She is a current MPH Candidate at the Columbia University Mailman School of Public Health and a Research Assistant at the Columbia University School of Nursing. She has been the recipient of many academic awards and has been involved in a wide range of research.

Faalik Zahra is a recent graduate from the University of Cincinnati who studied neuroscience and journalism. She has always had a strong inclination towards writing and sharing stories which have led her to pursue a journalism degree as well as founding an online media portal, Bearcat Voice. As a Senior Contributor, Faalik combines her passion for writing and her interest in medicine to work on educating patients on different medical illnesses, procedures, and treatments.

THE INDEX

Index

A

Aaliya Anaya, 175
Abigail Arient, 175
Access of Healthcare at the End of Life, 145
Access to Care, 30, 93
Accessibility to Nutritious Food, 26
Accessing Healthcare as a Nonbinary or Transgender Individual, 71
Addressing biases in healthcare, 74
Administrative Support Staff, 40
Administrators, 3, 19, 44
Adverse Childhood Experiences, 60
Age of Majority, 115
Age of the Patient, 142
Airiana Michelle Davis, 176
Allied Health Professions, 37
AMBULATORY CARE CENTERS, 51, 55
American College of Healthcare Executives, 11
American Culture, 25
American Dental Association, 12
American Hospital Association, 11
American Medical Association, 11
American Nursing Association, 11
Anat Ferleger, 177
Anooshka Shukla, 180
Are Healthcare Facilities Meeting Patient Expectations, 56
Artificial Nutrition and Hydration Near the End of Life, 147
Assisted Living Communities, 52

B

Balance issues, 130
Bansari Kheni, 177
Bansi H. Kakadiya, 177
Barriers in Communication, 155
Basic Inequities of Access to Healthcare - Men and Women, 67
Beth Duffy, 19
Birth to 12 Years Old, 110
Birth to Adolescence, 3, 110
Bridging the Gap Using Cultural Competency, 64

INDEX

Burnout, 52

C
Capacity, 137
Centers for Disease Control and Prevention (CDC), 46
Christopher R. Westfall, DMD, 16
Clinical Support Staff, 40
Cognitive Decline, 129
Common Health Issues That Senior-Aged Patients Face, 128
Communication Between Patient and Provider Is Essential, 155
Community and Social Context of the Patient, 140
Confidentiality and the Adolescent Patient, 113
Cost of Living, 29
Courtney Pokallus, 179
Culture of care and communication, 97

D
Danielle Ofri, MD, PhD, 15
Data collection and analysis, 75
De'Andre Alexander, 174
Decision to Move the Patient to Hospice and the Reasonable Expectations, 149
Defining Patient Centered Care, 10, 96
Dima Bischoff-Hashem, 176

Diverse health care teams, 75
Do Expectations Differ Based on The Social Determinants of Health, 139
Dwight McBee, 20

E
Economic Security, 29
Economic Stability of the Patient, 144
Education of a Healthcare Administrator, 44
Education of the Patient, 139
Educational Access and Patient Health Outcomes and Trends, 63
Effect of Adverse Childhood Experiences on Health, 61
Effect of Physical Environments, 58
Electronic Medical Records, 53
Emelia Behnan, 175
End of Life, 3, 135–136
Essential Roles of the Support Staff, 41
Evaluating the Care We Receive, 22

F
Faalik Zahra, 180
Fiduciary Relationship and Durable Power of Attorney, 136
Finding a Doctor Who Accepts Medicare, 131

INDEX

Finding the Right Administrator When You Need One, 49
Five Dimensions of Access, 94
Food and Drug Administration (FDA, 46

G

Gender Bias, 69
Gender Bias Against Women in Healthcare, 69
Gender of the Patient, 141

H

Having a Healthcare Professional in Your Social Circle, 90
Healthcare Facilities, 3
Healthcare Facilities, 51
Healthcare Facilities in Low-Income Neighborhoods, 86
Healthcare Marketplace, 116
Heart Disease, 129
Hospice Care Facilities, 52
Housing, Neighborhood, and Physical Environment, 28
How Administrators Impact Patient Centered Care, 47
How are Middle Age Patients Treated as Patients, 122
How Common Patient Complaints and Concerns Affect Patient Centered Care, 41
How Do the Social Determinants of Health Affect Access to Care, 95
How Do the Social Determinants of Health Affect Senior Care, 133
How Does Access to Care Impact Patient Centered Care, 98
Hugo Amador, 174

I

I Am a Patient, 169
Impact of a Patient's Access to Healthcare, 93
Impact of a Patient's Education, 60
Impact of a Patient's Gender, 67
Impact of a Patient's Social Circle, 89
Impact of a Patient's Socioeconomic Status, 76
Impact of Communication, 153
Impact of Corporate Medicine, 3, 161
Impact of Health insurance on Health Care, 77
Impact of Health Literacy on Navigating the Health System, 63
Impact of Health Literacy on Patient Centered Care, 62
Impact of Self-Determination on Food Consumption, 104

iii

Impact of Self-Determination on Reproductive Rights, 103
Impact of the Right to Self-Determination, 101
Impact of Where a Patient Lives, 82
Impact of Where a Patient Lives, 3
Implementing Patient Centered Care, 48
Importance of Patient-Provider Relationship, 154
Improving Seniors' Experiences at the Doctors, 134
Influence of Providers on Patient Centered Care, 39
Is Patient Centered Care Being Practiced, 168
Issue of Vaccinations, 106
Issues Seniors Face in Accessing Patient-Centered Care, 131

J
Juhi Patel, 179
Julianna Celestin, 176

L
Life Cycles of the Patient, 8
Lindsay Tobey, OTR/L, 13
Logan Nester, DPT, 17
Long-Term Care Facilities, 54

M
Major Decisions that Must Be Made at the End of Life, 146
Mason La Fleur, 178
Medical Miracles, 111
Medicare, 126
Meeting the Expectations of Patients: The Perspective of a Palliative Care Nurse, 148
Mental Health Providers, 39
Michael Cahill, LNHA, 19
Michelle Powell, 179
Middle Age, 3, 120

N
National Institutes of Health (NIH, 70
Not Having a Healthcare Professional in Your Social Circle, 90
Nursing Homes, 52

O
Occupational Therapist, 37
Olivia Arkell, 175
Oral health problems, 130
Osteoarthritis and Osteoporosis, 130

P
Palliative Sedation, 147
Patient Centered Care, 6
Patient Centered Care, 3
Patient Expectations, 55

INDEX

Patient Experience for the Homeless, 84
Patient Experience in Urban Areas, 82
Patient or Profit, 6
Patient Self-Determination Act, 101
Patient Self-Determination Act, 136
Patient's Access to Healthcare, 3
Patient's Education, 3
Patient's Gender, 3
Patient's Social Circle, 3
Patient's Socioeconomic Status, 3
Patient-Provider Relationship, 153
Patient-Provider Relationships Improve Healthcare Facilities, 159
patients actively participating in their own medical treatment, 96
Patients Prioritizing Choices, 80
Paul Kaloostian, M.D, 15
Pharmacist, 37
Physical Therapist, 38
Physician Assistant, 36
Physicians, 33
Picker Institute, 12
Presence of Healthcare Corporations, 162
Primary Care Provider, 94
Provider/Patient Communication, 3
Providers, 3, 13, 33
Providers Communicating with Low Health Literacy Patients, 158

R

Reasonable Expectations of a Patient in a Facility, 53
Reasonable Expectations of the Family at End of Life, 138
Reasonable Expectations of the Patient, 138
Regina Rush, 180
Resolving the Conflicts for the Sake of Better Patient Centered Care, 43
Respiratory Diseases, 131
Right of Self-Determination, 3, 136
Riham Alwaely, 174
Robert H. Kieserman, 178
Role of Culture on the Social Determinants, 25
Role of the Nurse, 35
Role of the Primary Care Provider, 94

S

Self-Determination and Compliance with Treatment Plans, 105
Self-Determination in Healthcare, 101
Senior Years, 3, 126

INDEX

Social Determinants of Health, 3
Social Determinants of Health and the Right to Self-Determination, 108
Socioeconomic Status, 76
Socioeconomic Status and Access to Healthcare, 76
Speech-Language Pathologist, 38
Strategies for Improving Healthcare Communication, 156
Substitution, 75
Supermarket Distance and Food Swamps, 27
Support Staff, 3, 40
Supportive health care environments, 97

T

Tasfia Wahid, 180
Teen Years to Young Adulthood, 113
Telehealth: Bridging the Gap Using Technology, 65
Training opportunities, 75
Transportation, 31
Traveling to Doctor's Appointments, 133
Treatment Plans and Prescription Drug Costs, 79
Two Major Types of Support Staff, 40

U

Use of Medications, 104

V

Vision and Hearing Loss, 131

W

Where Patients Gain Their Knowledge of Healthcare, 89
Who We Socialize With Can Impact Our Perceptions of Healthcare Delivery, 91
Withholding and Withdrawing Nonbeneficial Medical Interventions, 147
Women Access the Healthcare System More Than Men, 69
World Health Organization (WHO), 46

Y

Young Adult Demographic, 117
Young Adults, 3, 117
Yu-Tung Lu, 179

Made in the USA
Coppell, TX
30 May 2023